APPEARANCE VS. REALITY:

Bringing Forth the Opaque Effects of Traumatic Brain Injury (Tbi) into a Visual Experience

By Sandra Steranko

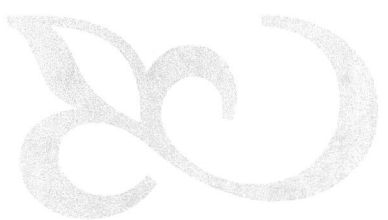

Interior and cover design by Ana Baird
www.AnaBananaCreations.com
Cover image © Marco Antonio Fdez/Dollar Photo Club

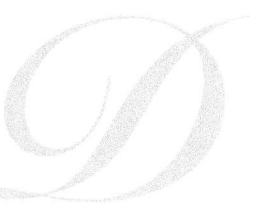

Dedicated to all traumatic brain injury (TBI) survivors and their supporters, along with the doctors and therapists who treat us with special care. Personally dedicated to my friends and family who have stood by me through the highs and lows, and to my biggest cheerleaders and supporters, Mom and Dad. Dad, I am sorry you didn't have the chance to see this finished. Even so, I know you are proud of me, as I am of you. This is especially for you.

Joseph Anthony Steranko
1936-2014

Table of Contents

Introduction

First and foremost, thank you for taking the time to read what I have passionately written. I am not medically trained in psychology nor in neuropsychology. All of my words are my interpretations from my own personal experiences. The words manifest from my heart and soul. My passion to write this book was conceived from my ongoing struggles with difficulty in understanding my personal experiences, the opaque challenges, and how others have reacted (or not known how to react) to the "reality" of the recovery/discovery process due to my traumatic brain injury (TBI). These are my thoughts, ending with hindsight after undergoing brain surgery—surgery that was secondary to life-threatening, uncontrollable, nocturnal epileptic seizures.

My purpose is to share my own journey so that patients (survivors) and their supporters may acquire understanding of the reality of TBI. Here I bring awareness into the recovery/discovery process of a survivor, awareness that will aid all in understanding the opaque recovery and effects resulting from TBI. In the end, my story grants a profound perception into the complexities of TBI recovery. Every moment of recovery presents a new discovery of experiences, beginning with the immediate effects, then continuing throughout the recovery/discovery process. I'll be frank: the healing process from a TBI is not a common rehabilitation from a common injury. For this reason, I am thankful for your interest in the reality, for wanting to understand the opaqueness.

Welcome, TBI survivors. I hope to support you with the encouragement, inspiration, and comfort you seek through the difficult times. I also have ambitions to make your personal experiences and challenges less burdensome and stressful through your recovery/discovery process. I offer you and your supporters a mental image of the difficult challenges and bizarre experiences you may encounter. Most importantly, I am writing so that you will know that you are not alone! Times of feeling isolated are inevitable. Please know that I am with you through my words.

Thank you, TBI supporters, for your interest. I wish to enlighten you from a survivor's perspective. At times, your efforts in helping and consoling will become challenging as well. You may sense that a survivor needs help, but you won't know the reason why or how you can give that help. You, too, will have moments of feeling confused or helpless. Loved ones particularly may become frightened. Please know that by sharing my experiences, I'm offering you the guidance and answers that I learned from them. I'm here for you, also.

Although this book focuses on my epileptic seizures, followed by my brain surgery, any type of TBI is complex, unique, delicate, and personal. I strongly believe any survivor acquiring these challenges can relate to portions of my journey in some way. My desire is to help you prepare for what you might be confronted with. What I am writing is not meant to sound scary or to be overly dramatic. It is meant to be straightforward and helpful. After all, if you are like me, you also choose to know all possible outcomes. Then you can prepare to confront them with vigor.

Some differences exist among those with TBI, differences in regard to the cause, location, and severity of the injury. Without dismissing them, I must note that there are also a few commonalities, the most prominent being that the recovery from *any* TBI remains mostly mental. To use my own phrase so that others can understand, "TBI is a mental dismemberment, *not* a physical one!" Therefore, "our" recovery/discovery is invisible or opaque while we heal. We are continually misperceived.

What is different across "our" population are the mental experiences. Some survivors may have none, while for others, they may be severe. What will not differ is that portions of your challenges will go unseen by the average onlooker. This is no fault of theirs. Not much has been published bringing forth the *reality* of the recovery from and the challenges of TBI and placing these challenges into a visual experience. The result has been an absence of knowledge that would allow others to be enlightened . . . until now.

Some of my challenges and those of my supporters might have been lessened or avoided if we had had more awareness with reality, both pre-op and post-op. Please don't misunderstand me. My fantastic doctors did their best to help me prepare within their scope of practice, meaning testing, medication, and surgery. What they could not help me prepare for was what I would mentally endure. Living in the spectrum of "appearance vs. reality" has led me to the conclusion that I *must* write this book! I must share my challenging journey in order to help others! Everyone needs to understand that TBI is not a superficial wound. It takes place in the core of our being. It originates from within.

Here is a pertinent example I encountered often when I no longer needed my walker or cane.

When someone I knew saw me, they would ask how I was doing. In my delayed and diffluent speech, I would say, "It has been a long struggle, with more hurdles to overcome."

Their reaction? "Really? Well, you look fine, so you must be doing fine."

"I have a mental dismemberment, not a physical one," I would repeatedly respond. "Of course I look fine."

> *A large portion of TBI survivors are living examples of appearance vs. reality. To put it into context, we can relate to the misguided judgment of an appearance from centuries ago. Man once believed the sun revolved around the Earth because that's how it appeared to the naked eye, but we know from space exploration that the belief of appearance was false. In reality, it is the Earth that revolves around the sun.*

After having to relive this uncomfortable confrontation regularly when cognitively able to make it out of the house, I've made it my mission to drill this particular philosophical perspective of mine into everyone's psyche. I do not feel or write this mission statement in anger. It's 100 percent frustration! Frustration is the common outcome a survivor will experience when deciphering and dealing with the complexities of having TBI, largely because common TBI effects are imperceptible.

Yes, the subtitle of my book is long. It reflects the length and complexity of the opaque challenges. From the start of my journey, I had two prominent focuses aside from healing. The first was to learn as much as I could from this experience. The second was to create a successful way to relay *what* I was feeling and going through emotionally and physically. My main objective at the time was to capture my mental challenges by taking what only I could see and experience, then placing them vividly on paper.

Personally, I learn, understand, and retain information best from pertinent examples, descriptions, and comparisons. Since my surgery, I have spent an abundance of time reflecting on and writing about how I feel, along with what I'm experiencing mentally and physically. Then one morning I awoke with this thought: *How can I successfully describe it to others?* How could I transform what I have been self-taught into visual experiences, I wondered, thus allowing the majority of individuals and my supporters to understand what they could not see. My answer was to write this book. It also answered my pre-operation question: "Why me, my Lord Jesus Christ?"

Keeping my fellow TBI survivors in the forefront during my writing, I completely understand how overwhelming reading, mentally processing, and retaining information can be, not to mention the mental fatigue involved! For us, these activities can resemble "driving in the fog." One, we need to go slow. Two, we may have passed something without noticing it. Three, when we arrive at our destination, we are mentally spent. Even though this book remains the same as a typical nonfiction book in that it tells an enjoyable story, it is written in an atypical nonfiction format. This is my way of writing to accommodate my fellow TBI readers. The chapters need to remain short. I believe it will also be helpful to share my writing style to make *this* book more enjoyable for survivors to read.

I find comfort looking at things from a philosophical perspective. For instance, I say, "Brain surgery is not a quick fix. Brain surgery is a new beginning." Also, "Without a challenge, there is neither growth nor reward." It is enjoyable for me to create my own proverbs, such as "Expectations most commonly lead to frustration and disappointment. Inspiration can bring success and fulfillment to both." For the broad experiences, I try to simplify them within one word. The most frequent one I use in this book and in daily life is "unknown."

The concept of the unknown was created over time. As my journey continues, so do the experiences. Therefore, I have taken all of the unfamiliar surroundings, the uncertainty, the fear, the panic, and the cognitive unawareness up to this point and placed them into the unknown. In simplistic terms regarding the reality of our recoveries, most everything *is* unknown. From my personal enlightenment, I've concluded that recovery equals discovery. That is why these words are interchangeable for those with TBI.

My goal is to assist both TBI survivors and TBI supporters, and I hope that what I write will assist you in several ways: by helping you prepare if you're having surgery, by giving you foresight and understanding of possible experiences, and most importantly, by instilling positive thoughts during your recovery/discovery and throughout your opaque journey.

A few words about my writing style. I do not take TBI or its recovery lightly. However, I *do* write with a light heart, sprinkled with humor. I live and write with the belief that "humor heals." Trust that humor will assist you, as it has me, in overcoming some of the challenges and fears on your journey. I say, "Humor will bring light into your darkness." I also feel that through humor, the superficial wounds will heal much faster, easier, and with less self-pain. So feel free to laugh as much as you want as I share my experiences. It would be nice to have someone laughing *with* me, not just *at* me. Unfortunately, the latter does happen when it comes to TBI survivors. Some people just don't get it. I hope, for the sake of all of us, they soon will.

Lastly, in order to accommodate my fellow survivors, I will keep the book reader friendly. One way is by placing quotation marks around some of my creative thoughts and examples, like "Humor will bring light into your darkness." I will also be using subparagraphs when explaining my philosophies and vivid details when I begin to bring forth my encounters with the opaque, as I did in my explanation of appearance vs. reality. This way you can refer to them quickly if and when needed. I am confident that relaying my journey will assist you to better prepare, understand, and instill positive thoughts during your recovery and that my writing will aid you and your supporters throughout your personal journey.

By practicing the above methods, I have gained a greater knowledge and acceptance of my life, along with a positive attitude. I've also had rewarding outcomes when I've implemented all or some of them while enlightening my supporters and other individuals about the challenges I face.

Now that I've delved into the format and substance of the book (the not-so-fun-stuff), allow me to introduce myself on a personal basis. While I reach out to the survivors, I'd like you to recognize more of who I am through sharing my thought processes, along with examples of my personality. This is my way of bonding with the readers and survivors. In addition, I'll be sharing my viewpoint of myself, how I lived my life prior to brain surgery, and how I am struggling to live the same afterward. Trust me. This will be fun to read. As a tease, let me add this: some people say I was "messed up" *before* having surgery.

ಐಐಐ

To begin, I consider myself independent. I'm very self-sufficient. I try to figure things out on my own. Because of my pride, I rarely ask for help, and I prefer to do things my own way on my own terms. Others call me stubborn. Can you believe that?

I'm a private person who respects other people's privacy. It is not often that I ask or answer personal questions. Being an introvert also, my thoughts and feeling are that, if someone wishes for me to know something personally, then they'll tell me. In exchange, if I wish for

viii

someone to know something personal about me, then I'll tell them. Therefore, I've never been one to stand by the "water cooler" and partake in gossip. As a result, others see me as a "loner" to put it politely. My response? R-E-S-P-E-C-T.

I'm a *very* organized individual. I live by "a place for everything and everything in its place." My closet displays the color wheel in subcategories, from sleeveless shirts to long-sleeved sweaters. What my brother-in-law, Bill, finds the most humorous (or disturbing) is that I rotate my set of steak knives. Who wouldn't want them to wear evenly? With that reasoning, I rotate everything in the house. When I take on a task, I prepare two steps ahead, each having multiple contingency plans.

Those who have witnessed my organizational skills label me "Type A with a dash of OCD." Well . . . maybe. My neuropsychologist at the time, Dan, read this as a draft. He half-jokingly questioned if I was being treated for the correct issue! This is a good time for you to laugh, because *I'm* laughing. I warned you I was messed up prior to surgery. Although I possess these quirks, overall, I *am* a laid-back person. Honestly! With exceptions.

In some areas of life, my motivation is fierce. My comfort zone is not being average. I strive to be above average. If I feel I've failed myself or let someone down, I try to make it up somewhere else. Others perceive me as an overachiever. Really? When I have connections or responsibilities to someone or something, I am loyal and try my best. If over time I concede it's not working, then I cut my losses and move on. For example, I once packed what I could fit in my car and moved across the country. Some individuals would consider me a quitter for doing that. Wrong again. I was fearless!

My favorite professor, Ellen Meyer Gregg, who holds a bachelor's and a master's degree in speech and language pathology and a doctorate in communication disorders and speech science, summed me up the best. She described me most eloquently. During our correspondence after surgery, Ellen said I have *tenacity*. Thank you, Ellen! This is one of the nicest compliments I've ever been given. In addition, it confirmed how I coped when my illness wouldn't cease, then reinforced my inner strength to take on the challenges awaiting after surgery.

There are a few items about me which are non-debatable. For example, I'm determined to be a survivor. There are many choices in our lives. The following are a few of the choices I've made. I've chosen *not* to be a victim in my lifetime! I don't give up without a fight. Nor do I willingly settle for less. I refuse to surrender to anyone or anything! I meet every challenge head-on. These choices were an asset after my initial battle with epileptic seizures. Thankfully, my tenacity and humor have carried me through.

So please, while you read, laugh when you feel like it, enjoy my story, and take from my words and journey whatever will help you and your supporters. To show my rebellious side by writing a cliché, I say, "It can be a bumpy ride on the road to your recovery." I hope to help you to some degree to make sure your bum doesn't hurt too badly during your journey. On that note . . . buckle up and enjoy the reality throughout my wild ride with TBI, beginning with a chapter about my seizures. Enjoy!

Author's Note

*N*ot only am I bringing you into the challenges of TBI through my experiences by examples, but you will be experiencing it for yourself in a real, developmental way as you continue reading. As I continued writing, my cognition was becoming clearer. This is reflected in my writing style, which was also becoming clearer. I wanted to give you the full encompassing experience however I could. Enjoy it as I did.

ಐ

Chapter 1

Battleground with Seizures

*T*he initial encounters with my seizures were masked by the darkness of night. I had no intuition of what was taking place as I slept. When I'd awaken, being unaware a battle had taken place, my physical being would feel as if it had been hit by a truck . . . literally. Every muscle in my body was tight, achy, and weak. It was a challenge to gather what little strength and energy I had remaining, just to make it through a normal day. In addition, I strove to make it a successful one.

In the morning, my head felt heavy and would be pounding from deep within. During the night as I would seize, the seizures were transforming the anatomy of my brain into a bowling ball. This is how it felt while moving afterward.

A minute movement of my head caused my brain to have the sensation of a bowling ball rolling around inside my head, stopping only when making abrupt contact with the skull. The simple

> *task of brushing my teeth would cause it to roll*
> *from side to side, along with rolling backward and*
> *forward while I was brushing. When I would finish*
> *with a rinse, the rolling ball would stop by slam-*
> *ming into the front of my skull, causing me severe*
> *pain. The same sensation and pain repeated itself*
> *when I moved my head even slightly in any di-*
> *rection, from the time I began getting dressed to*
> *when I put on and tied my shoes.*

I tried taking precautions, such as brushing slower to lessen any head movement and vibrations. I even tried to keep my mouth level with the sink so I wouldn't have to tilt my head down. These precautions didn't help. Just the slightest movement opened up the longest alley for the bowling ball to roll down, picking up speed on the way to hitting the pins—my skull, of course, being the pins. If it had been a true game of bowling, my brain would have had a perfect score every time. Ouch!

I lived ignorant of the seizures for a while, until one night there was a witness to these battles. I had been hospitalized, and the doctor on call informed me I was having seizure activity. Unfortunately, there was no neurologist immediately available to examine me, so I waited and counted the days till the appointment.

In the meantime, by day my mind began to absorb what was happening. I was already a private person and an introvert, and now I no longer had any desire or confidence to be social outside of work or my home. By night, the battles continued. The seizures were giving me a beating mentally and physically. All of my physical strength and energy was spent during the nights, seizing.

Accompanying the pain caused by my nocturnal seizures was fear. Even the nights I was most tired, I would be afraid to fall asleep. After placing my head on my pillow, I could not refrain from wondering if this would be my last living moment. Would a seizure overtake me during the night while asleep? Would it cause me to swallow my tongue? After surviving the nights, I'd awaken with a swollen, bloody, chewed tongue. Even so, I chose to see it as a positive. I was given the gift of one more day.

Because I lived alone the majority of the time, my nights were solely spent between me and my seizures. I was at their mercy. This brought no comfort to my independence or relief from my taste of fear. My nocturnal seizures had become so overbearing that my quality of life had plummeted, and my physical safety became a major concern. Finally, my neurologist appointment was here! Now I should receive some answers and help, or so I hoped.

Our initial visit was the usual question-and-answer period. Then he ordered two tests: a standard MRI and an EEG while I slept for only a couple of hours. Upon our second visit, my "first" neurologist and I reviewed the results from the tests he had ordered. After the review, the cause for my nocturnal epileptic seizures was undetermined. Unfortunately in the seizure population, it is typical to have unknown causes. This answer was difficult for me to accept, but I didn't have the knowledge to challenge the doctor. Therefore, at the time I had to accept it. What happened next, though, had a different outcome.

He wrote a prescription and said, "I thought for sure

it was a tumor when you first came in. Take these meds and see how it goes." I'm paraphrasing, but his flippant response, lack of information, and convenient remedy were *not* acceptable to me. I asked the following question with sincerity: "When I begin to experience a precursor to a seizure, can I self-will the seizures to stop?" (In my case, the precursors were déjà vu disguised as dreams and rancid odors that would wake me up.) The doctor's inability to acknowledge my determination and unwillingness to settle passively had him respond with a chuckle. Therefore, I found a more helpful and empathetic neurologist.

With the sincerity and knowledge of my second neurologist, Allen Gee, MD, PhD, I experienced a period of time that was seizure-free. Dr. Gee and I believed we had the correct meds after several changes . . . until one night. From out of the darkness, my seizures returned with a vengeance. The changes in meds hadn't offered any permanent relief. The cause was still unknown.

My taste of fear turned into terror. The battle I had experienced upgraded to a civil war inside my brain. The seizures/enemies were encroaching deeper into my territory. Now this challenge became *more* personal. I felt that the seizures were trying to show that they had control over me. So . . . I *retaliated!*

Chapter 2

Stratagem

With the eruption of the civil war, I had to form a new defensive strategy. I needed to collect as much "intel" about my enemy as possible. I was on a mission to find more evidence about my seizures. No longer was I going to allow myself to be at their mercy. Nor was I any longer going to allow the "that's how it is" mentality to be an educated answer. I was in search of facts but didn't know where to begin.

Therefore, I asked myself six questions: Who is the enemy? My seizures. What are they? Nocturnal epileptic. When did they appear? Reappeared recently. Why? Can't be determined. How? Remains unknown. Where in the brain do they occur? That hasn't been explored thoroughly. That's it! This is where I'll begin! This will be my strategic move. Locate the source

I decided to find as many facts as I could specifically concerning "where" the seizures were originating from. In retaliation, I was going to find the intel as to the location of the enemies' base camp, where they lay in wait. Then I would strategize using those facts, thus creating a plan to become resilient in this war. Dr. Gee was willing to assist in any manner needed. He gave me the compass and direction.

The first quest for intel led me to Casper, Wyoming. My determination to prevail began with a long-term, video-monitored EEG. When I arrived at hospital admissions, I was mentally prepared for the average, five-day stay required for this test. *Ten* days later, due to the relentless seizing, I was discharged. Those ten days of physical and mental torture, though, gave me the advantage. I felt satisfied. Of course, I also felt sleep-deprived and weak, as if I'd been hit by a rig and dragged over rocks, but I was mostly satisfied.

As my seizures thought they were having a "non-medicated free-for-all" in the hospital, unbeknown to them, they were giving my scrutinizing neurologist, David Wheeler, MD, PhD, an abundance of intel. *Facts*, lots of facts! During my nightly slumbers, the seizures were out of control. My enemies thought *they* were in control. Thankfully, the plan to deceive them was working. Their every action was being recorded on paper and video. I graciously declined watching the video when asked. I was living it and didn't need to see it. I knew the hospital meant no disrespect, but it was just too soon. Anyway, the indeterminate data I had going into the hospital had become undeniable data by the time of my discharge.

Over the ten days of brutality, the seizures came closer to revealing the source of their activities, including how long and intense they would fight before returning to their base camp. We *now* knew the general location of their primary camp was in my right hemisphere. They had given the doctor and me the facts, facts that would be used to take out my enemies. At the time, I didn't realize how literal that sentence was.

You see, their hyperactivity and persistence made my case severe, so severe that it caused Dr. Wheeler to submit a referral package to Seattle, Washington, for further testing, with my consent. Depending on Seattle's findings, the most successful treatment could result in my having brain surgery to resect the "problem areas." Now my stratagem was in motion.

I hoped to go to Harborview to learn more. I felt very fortunate because I believed Harborview to be the best research hospital for seizures. One of the many reasons for my belief was that the doctors and staff were very thorough in finding detailed answers. Therefore, after Dr. Wheeler told me the plan, my chest felt lighter, and I could breathe deeper. I thought to myself, *As an individual who's a stickler for details and perfection, I'm confident this will be a perfect union!*

During the time my referral package was under review in Seattle, I was home trying to regain control. It seemed as though my elongated stay in the hospital had empowered the seizures. Trying yet another seizure med didn't suppress their activity. On the contrary, I was either waking up sick in the middle of the night or oversleeping from the physical/mental abuse that was occurring. Soon after this development, I received a call from Harborview.

Carol, the lovely lady from the office of specialist John Miller, MD, had called. She relayed that my referral packet was presented at an epilepsy conference. Hence, Dr. Miller wanted to meet with me for a consultation. (My mental picture was like a television series at the time.) Along with his appointment, I would be scheduled for a series of additional tests. Suffering from the recent activities, I eagerly asked if this meant I was a candidate for surgery. Carol told me it was not a quick decision to make, that there were sequential steps the doctors and staff would be taking so the hospital could make an informed evaluation for a final decision, just as they wanted me to make an informed decision. Gosh, I was so impressed with this medical establishment!

Carol was also straightforward that this would be the first of possibly several visits. "Would you be able to commit to this if you accept?" she asked.

Without missing a beat, my expressive language said, "Yes, please. I'm very grateful." Internally, I thought, *Expletive, yeah!*

Near the end of our conversation, Carol said she would be mailing me a detailed itinerary. This would include the dates, times, tests with detailed instructions, the doctors/specialists I would be meeting with, and a map of the hospital and university. I told you this would be a perfect union! Thank goodness for the maps, too. I can read a map but have never mastered reciting my right from left. It has always been either "Turn your way" or "Turn my way." At the close of the phone call, Carol asked if I had any more questions.

Just one. "How many days should I plan for, so I can make the appropriate flight and hotel reservations?"

Her response . . . five days.

Oh boy, I had heard that before.

After taking a day to process my up-and-coming adventure, I realized I could not "go this one alone," independently as I would prefer and as I had done in Casper.

I understood that I needed someone to go through this process with me, someone I deemed trustworthy to sit in on the appointments with the medical team. I needed someone who knew my medical history, someone I could confide in and with whom I would feel comfortable sharing the new information. Most importantly, under the circumstances, I needed a person who also preferred to choose humor over fear and stress. With that last requirement, my sister, Sonia, came to mind. She, too, likes to keep things lighthearted.

When I called Sonia to invite her to take the trip to Seattle, she did not hesitate. It was set. She and I would meet at the Seattle airport. I told her Dr. Miller's office would be mailing me the itinerary and maps. Referring to my right-left issue, Sonia laughed at how much good that would do for us. She said she would spring for a GPS. After that shared laugh, I was so happy to have asked her and also relieved and grateful she had accepted.

ॐ

Chapter 3

Something to Ponder

*T*he morning arrived for my first adventure to Seattle. An adventure is how I was looking at it, though my nerves were on high alert. I had my itinerary, so I understood what to expect literally. It was the gray area, the findings of my tests, that had me troubled. Trying to keep my nerves calm, I kept reminding myself that it was all routine. The doctors and technicians did this every day. My tests would be no different. This self-reasoning kept my nerves in check till the flight left.

As the plane ascended into the clouds, I tried to keep my body grounded. I let my mind wander with random thoughts. At first, they were about simple things. *Did I make the bed? Did I lock the door when I left?* But those thoughts only masked my anxiety. Then my thoughts went deeper. I let myself grip what lay ahead. My philosophical side came out, and I thought about the human brain. I could think of nothing else at this time.

In essence, the human brain is enigmatic. The human brain may have a common blueprint as to where the sections are physically located, but that is the only definite commonality. How it functions is unique for every individual. An analogy I created to aid in understanding this concept is as follows.

It could be said that healthy human hands have a patent. All humans know how a healthy hand looks and functions. For instance, your phalanges, the bones in your fingers, move. You can use your thumb to pinch. All ten fingers can be used to play the piano, and you can transform an open hand into a fist. Basically, the functions of healthy human hands are consistent in the human population, and they are all physical functions.

If a part is broken, it most commonly can be located with precision by the use of an x-ray or MRI machine. Then common steps can be taken to repair it, whether by using a hard cast or pins to reset it and put it back into its proper place. Rods can replace certain bones when severely broken. The recovery is visual and tangible. One knows how it should look and function.

But for the healthy human brain, there is no consistent functional blueprint. Also, nothing can be replaced. The brain is the only mental functioning part of the human body and is incomparable to all other parts. Mental function is unseen, intangible, unpredictable, and never the same between two people. We are all "hardwired." Science may tell us what areas functions begin in, but where those wires cross and connect can be different. Therefore, the human brain cannot have one patent for everycne.

Even the brains that are put into categories for diagnosis, such as Alzheimer's, autism, or epilepsy, are different. The human brain can have only one patent per individual. If something in the brain is "broken," the source of the problem might be too complicated to be found with only an x-ray or MRI. Just knowing where to begin looking may be difficult to determine. When the source of the problem is found, remedies may be limited. If something needs to be removed, there is nothing to replace it. In the case of the human brain, each brain is unique and may never be fully discovered.

What will they discover about my brain in Seattle? I wondered as the flight continued on.

Chapter 4

Exploration of My Mind

*S*onia and I met at the Seattle airport as expected. It was the day before my first round of scheduled appointments began. Our first stop, of course, coffee! Next, we located our luggage and rental car. Then we were off to find a grocery store and finally our hotel. Yes, we had the GPS. In my defense, I heard "recalculating" more than once, Sonia.

By the time we settled into our suite and ate, it was late. By my standards, we had to awaken at o'dark hundred. Our first appointment was for my first scheduled test, 3 Tesla MRI, a more detailed image MRI. Then we would meet separately with neurologist Dr. Miller and neurosurgeon Dr. Ojemann. The previous short night and long day were hard on me mentally, as mental fatigue is for TBI survivors. I certainly don't recall having had trouble falling asleep on this particular night, but I remember being brought to by my sister. From her room above, Sonia could hear my alarm going off. She came in to wake me up. Yes, I was seizing. Perhaps I was more stressed and fatigued than I had thought.

We successfully recalculated to my first appointment. While my head was being examined, Sonia located where Dr. Miller's office was in the next building we had to travel to. She returned as I was finishing redressing. After I was done, we were on our way to meet Dr. Miller. In addition to a consultation, Dr. Miller performed a physical exam, reviewed my seizure history, and went over the risk factors involved. In regard to my meetings with the doctors, I am only going to share what is pertinent to this book.

My first and lasting impression of Dr. Miller was that of a kind and gentle man. He showed the perfect balance of professionalism and humanity. Now that we were in a private setting, he was able to give me more understanding of how the candidate process works. He expanded on the phone conversation I had with Carol.

My referral package from Dr. Wheeler was presented at an epilepsy conference. After review, the conference recommended that I could be a possible surgical candidate, though I first needed to come to Seattle for the tests I've already noted. Once I concluded the tests and meetings, my case would be presented at conference again. If there was clear localizing info, only then would consideration be given to having me return for surgical treatment. I concurred with the process entirely.

Following this conversation, he cut to the chase. "When was your last seizure?"

"This morning," I replied.

Sonia went over the event she had witnessed. I believe he raised his eyebrows before taking more notes. Our informative consultation was almost over. It ended with the risk factors. First, possible death. I was living with that burden every night before closing my eyes. Second, about a one percent chance of stroke. Personally, I felt that would be less debilitating than what I was currently living with. Dr. Miller knew I was seeing Dr. Ojemann next. In that appointment, Dr. Ojemann would be going over my morning's test with me.

Sonia and I were halfway through our first day of tests and appointments, with several grueling ones to come, and it was already becoming overwhelming for me mentally. On the positive side, even though the tests were long, they were very interesting. Our country's advancements in medical technologies are just amazing! The detailed images the technologies now produce are spectacular! I also appreciated that the tests I was having done were noninvasive and didn't ask personal questions as nurses do, questions such as "How tall are you? How much do you weigh?"

The nurse who asked me those questions didn't appreciate or find the humor in me asking her for clarification. "What the scale reads or my driver's license?"

The doctors on the other hand, were much more personable and lighthearted. This leads me to our next appointment, one which I will never forget. Dr. Ojemann might never have forgotten it either. Our first encounter!

As Sonia and I waited in the office for Dr. Ojemann to arrive, she asked me if I was nervous. "No, not yet," I said, uncertainly. Our purpose for the appointment was to look at and go over my earlier 3 Tesla MRI, with the objective of finding out if there was correlation within the localizing areas. I knew I was one step closer to finding answers to my previous objective of finding the source, along with the new objective: brain surgery. I believe my palms were a little damp. It could have been from either the anticipation or Seattle's fall weather.

Dr. Ojemann entered the room. You could tell he was all business, but he had a calming presence and a nice smile. He sat next to me, and Sonia sat on the medical table behind us. It was showtime! He brought up the images of my brain on his screen. We were reviewing them as he explained what all the colors and dark spots meant. Then suddenly, Sonia gasped. "Oh my!"

Dr. Ojemann looked at her with concern and asked if everything was okay.

Sonia replied, "Yes, I'm just excited to see she has a brain!"

Oh, aren't big sisters great! We all had a good laugh, again bringing the light into the darkness, which was good timing.

All the tests, going back to my video EEG, had produced interrelated results. It was evident that my seizures were originating in my right temporal lobe, and I had severe damage in some areas, thus causing the appointment to become more serious. Dr. Ojemann talked with me about the same risk factors as Dr. Miller had. I acknowledged them, said I understood, and asked to continue with the process. The trip had now transferred from exploring my mind with the possibility of surgery to hypothetically scheduling my brain surgery. Relying on his medical expertise and experience, Dr. Ojemann put me on the calendar while the process went through its formalities. He spent a great deal of time in our non-rushed appointment explaining the surgery and showing Sonia and me what he planned to resect (remove).

The procedure would begin with the removal of my

whole right temporal lobe (a temporal lobectomy). Then he would tailor layers off my right hippocampus. I think of *tailored* as a medically sophisticated (hoity-toity) term Dr. Ojemann used for *shaved*. Dr. Ojemann explained that before he made any resections, he wanted proof from three different tests showing the same problem locations and abnormalities from several weeks prior to possibly the day before surgery. I thought that was justifiable and found it comforting. We had just reviewed my first test. I was scheduled the next day for a PET study and neuropsychological testing. Did I mention that I did very well on this one?

Some people might have felt animus toward the doctors for ordering the numerous tests I'd had and would have. My perspective going through this long process reverted to my theory of the brain and how unique, delicate, and special the brain is. An individual needs to respect what they have and have a doctor who shares that respect! Therefore, find a doctor and/or neurosurgeon who is willing to take additional time to order more than one test. Don't think of it as the institution trying to make money. Think of it as the doctors being vigilant, cautious, having your best interests at heart, and most importantly, giving *you* the *best* care, which you deserve.

Find comfort as I did when they take you and their profession seriously. Also, be reassured when they're doing due diligence to make certain that what they plan to do to your brain is correct. What is resected can never be replaced. Brain surgery is unlike resetting a broken hand. Brain surgery cannot be readjusted later. I very much appreciated the doctors for being so thorough. At the time, it gave me more trust, comfort, and a greater probability for success.

In addition to the doctors possessing these qualities, the patient needs to arrive at the appointments prepared. As a patient, don't carry doom and gloom with you to the doctors. Instead, carry a list of questions. Take the time you have before your appointments to come up with as many questions as you can think of. Also, ask your family and supporters if they have any. During stressful times, occasionally the most obvious questions are overlooked. For example, while I was busy asking Dr. Ojemann about dementia and such, Sonia chimed in. "How long is the average surgery and hospital stay?" *Duh*, Sandra. Great question, Sonia.

Most importantly, don't be hesitant to ask anything. Remember, the only irrelevant question is the question not asked. By this I mean, don't be afraid to ask anything. Ignorance is not bliss. On the part of you or your supporters, ignorance will only make it harder on yourself later. Not asking questions allows more open space for the unknown to creep in.

So to help get you started, here are several questions I thought of before and after my initial visit: How many surgeries have you performed? What are the most and least common short-term and long-term effects? What are the most common feelings and reactions someone has when waking up after surgery? What is your definition of a successful surgery? (In my personal case, I believe it was that I made it off the table—no joking here.) Is there one thing in particular that will help my transition when going home? Lastly, is there anything I should have asked that I didn't? Encourage the doctors to think of a pertinent question, too!

For those who incessantly use the Internet to find information independently, please proceed with caution! A lot of information can be found, but it cannot replace a one-on-one with an experienced professional. Some information you read might be vague, false, misleading, or not in context. For example, online articles are prominent that say language is stored in the left temporal lobe, therefore leading the reader to assume that having a right temporal lobectomy wouldn't affect the patient's language. Having learned this while studying speech-language pathology, I concur that some language is stored in the left temporal lobe. However, my personal experience after surgery can back up that not all of your language is stored in the left. Some is stored in the right. A statement that "most language" is located in the left temporal lobe would be more accurate and non-misleading to the reader. It's not only about semantics. It's about reality.

Skipping ahead for a moment to prove the importance of my thought, let me say that a misleading or out-of-context detail such as this can bring frustration and confusion to you and your supporters. One of my delayed outcomes was acquired aphasia (disfluent speech), with a decrease in word retrieval and cognitive processing. A dear friend tried to talk with me by phone several days after surgery. She could not grasp the concept that I was having difficulty with my language because "The Internet said . . ." Please don't misunderstand me. I am grateful that someone cared enough to take the initiative to try to understand and prepare for what I would be like after surgery. Thank you for trying and caring. What made it frustrating and difficult for both of us was that the online information had been perceived as the gospel. My point is this: technology cannot replace doctors and personal experiences when it comes to answers and explanations. In essence, the human brain is opaque. In my friend's defense, sure, language may be "stored" in one place even though retrieval might go through several channels. I also suffered a mild stroke, but I'll get to that later.

In hindsight, there was one resource I wish I had had deeper access to: the neuropsychologist. I only met the one who'd administered my neuropsychological test, and that was the extent of our visit. Now I strongly believe the neuropsychologist's educational training would have given me more realistic expectations for my recovery and the experiences I have since encountered. Of course, the doctor and neurosurgeon mentioned a few possibilities, although it was not in their scope of practice to go in-depth. Nevertheless, having a discovery session with a neuropsychologist, I now know, would have been a valuable asset to have had, beginning from my waking moments and continuing on for years, especially for a person such as myself, someone who needs concrete information and understanding.

Examples of questions I would have asked would be: Why don't I recognize my face in the mirror? What part of the brain is affected to make this happen? Is there a specific brain process for visual recognition? Even though it's stored in the right temporal lobe, will it come back, adapt, or reprogram itself? Examples for the supporters would be: What cognitive abilities will she need help with? Beyond talking slower, what can we do to be supportive and not cause any surprises? I strongly recommend that anyone who is preparing for brain surgery or who has acquired TBI, along with their supporters, talk with a neuropsychologist.

To the neuropsychologists, I firmly encourage you to make yourselves accessible to be spoken with. You are desperately needed through the entirety of pre-op and recovery, not only for the patients, but also for their family and supporters. As a whole, we need your understanding and knowledge of what TBI patients experience mentally. Most importantly, we need the knowledge and coping skills you have to offer to help everybody through the rough and frustrating periods. *Please*, I ask of you with sincere compassion, make yourselves known and available to TBI survivors and their supporters.

Okay, moving on.

Thankfully, this trip to Seattle was balanced between fun and anxiety. In addition to Sonia's role as sister, supporter, extra pair of ears, and chauffeur, she was also my comic relief. For instance, I felt so guilty for taking her time away from her husband, Bill; my nephew, Tyler; and her demanding job. Sonia was able to sense that I felt as if I were placing a burden on her. She told me, "Hey, don't worry about it! I've always wanted to vacation in Seattle! Never been here!"

Thanks, Sonia. Happy I could help you in return!

A personal piece of insight into my family is that most of us enjoy playing cards and board games. Sonia and I are notorious for bringing out the Scrabble board. The funny part is I have always been a terrible speller. Since adolescence, I've practiced, "When in doubt, add an E at the end." Sonia continues to remind me, along with others, so graciously, that I used to spell *with* W-H-

I-T-H or W-I-T-H-E. Yes, I'm aware that is bad. As a result of my terrible spelling, Sonia loves to play this game with me, first, because she has a good laugh. Secondly, she usually wins. In my defense, I tell her that if we had a broader dictionary that included my words, she wouldn't win as often! Nevertheless, we always have fun time mixed with quality time together. So, after the grueling, stressful, and emotional days of tests and appointments, we would sit down to play a couple of games to banish the previous.

Finally it was time to pack up the game and our clothes. We would part ways at the airport in the morning. Sonia would return to a normal life in Denver. I would return to Cody and wait for a phone call. Would I be accepted or rejected for medical treatment? The conference had much information to scrutinize before a final decision would be made. Even though I was returning home (and on schedule this time), I felt as if my quality of life hung in the balance. Would I even survive to know the decision?

Chapter 5

Anticipation

After traveling home, the first thing I did was check the answering machine . . . nothing. This became a ritual when leaving the house for any length of time. It continued for about a week. One day while I was out, I felt the need to come home. There was no message, but shortly after I hung up my coat, the phone rang. It was Carol from Harborview. She pleasantly asked how I was. I told her no better. I was still living in fear, as the seizures persisted at night. Carol was calling to give me an answer. The answer was hope.

My case had been presented at the epilepsy conference. After the review, I was formally considered a surgical candidate. This news brought me overwhelming relief and excitement. With all the prevailing symptoms I'd been living with, I was looking forward to having brain surgery. Knowing I could have this surgery gave me hope for the possibility of a more normal than harmful life. Carol was mailing me a new itinerary.

When the call ended, the first thing I had to do was

calm my emotions and process what had just taken place. My second order of business was to contact family and close friends. In some cases I seemed to be the more positive person. Through no fault of their own, some individuals were still hung up on what had caused my seizures in the first place. For me, that question had become irrelevant a while ago. Now I needed to remain focused on what I had to do to survive and to get my quality of life back. I didn't even have time to be nervous or worried. I chose to not look in the past. Instead, I chose to place my focus and positive energy into being proactive. I achieved this by preparing for my "new beginning."

Once my surgery was confirmed, I had only a couple of weeks to prepare and to get my affairs in order. Luckily, I was an organized person. My organizational skills saved me time because I already had created a few lists I would need. This allowed me time to make additional ones. Not being sure how my memory recall would be after surgery, I triple-checked my spreadsheets that listed bills and their due dates and reviewed my calendar/planner, listing future appointments and deadlines along with any special dates. Then I logged all usernames and passwords, which I highly recommend. What I had overlooked and what would have helped me was writing basic instructions on how to operate anything mechanical, for example, the television remote, DVR, VCR, and the washer and dryer. In hindsight, it would have helped me, along with my parents, who would be staying with me after the surgery. The potential for problems when operating technology was vast.

The last list I wrote was for my sister to use after my operation. About this particular list, it was a list of people for Sonia to contact when I came out of surgery. My dear friend Laura reminded me the other day when talking that I drew a smiley face next to the names I considered to be my genuine friends, separating them from acquaintances as a precaution in case I forgot after surgery who I could trust. I told Laura, "I don't remember doing that, but it sure does sound like me." By indicating my close friends, I was preparing for any mental vulnerability I would have. Unfortunately, the list was useful because there were people who did try to take advantage of my vulnerability.

Not knowing how long or to what extent my inactivity would be after brain surgery, I also made a list of items to stock in my home, items I used most often or that I would feel uncomfortable having others get for me. The neurosurgeon had forewarned me that my head wound would be sensitive to the cold air for a time. Because my surgery was taking place in November, I was most certain that my outdoor activity when I returned to Wyoming would pose a challenge. Therefore, I purchased a piece of exercise equipment. Little did I know that I had foresight when ordering it. My original intention was to use it to replace walking outside in the cold. Its actual purpose turned out to be to aid my balance and help me learn to walk independently again. Good call, Sandra!

During this prep time, I continued to stay positive and focused. I was thinking and planning ahead to the best of my ability. What altered my demeanor was writing my living will. Reflecting back, I believe this was the moment when my personal stages of grief moved forward. When making the tough decisions required, I became *angry* and disquieted.

"Lord, I'm only thirty-six years old. Why?"

His answer to my quest was returned from the beginning: to find the answers and relay them to help others. I decided at that moment to hand my situation over to God. With my lists made, bags packed, and faith in heart, it was time to go.

⁋⁋⁋

Sonia and I were back in Seattle in our same suite. Two nights before my surgery and after I had had my final CT scan and functional MRI, we sat down to play our common game of Scrabble. Only this time, it wasn't common. It was our first quiet game. During the game, my wondering about the surgery began. My mind was racing with inner inquiry. *What will I or won't I remember? Who will I or won't I recognize? Will I be able to begin graduate school this summer? Overall, what will I be like? Will I still be me? Will I have my self-drive, intelligence, ability to remain independent? What challenges will I encounter?*

I was embarking on my journey through the "unknown frontier." My fearlessness was abandoning me, and the taste of fear was rising in my throat. It tasted sour.

Then Sonia said something during our game that changed my outlook and changed it to this day. "Hey, if your curly hair grows back straight and you can spell correctly, you could be a medical freaking marvel!"

The room became brighter the harder we laughed together. As a bonus, what she said gave me a goal. I would find satisfaction in being a medical marvel. Yeah, awesome! She took a quick picture of me the night before surgery to compare with after. I'm not there yet. My hair remains curly. I'm still trying to locate a dictionary that includes the spelling of my words. Even so, I'm dedicated to continuing to strive to reach my goal every day. Thanks again, Sonia. You're the best big sister!

The day before surgery, we picked Mom and Dad up from the airport. It was very emotional for all. Everyone has their own way of handling stress and fear. The way the situation developed, I was trying to comfort and reassure others that things would be all right, but I wasn't saying anything negative toward anyone. I know my family was there to support me. That's what matters most. I am eternally grateful and love them dearly for being there and for giving me the support I needed.

In hindsight, my advice to supporters is to remain calm. Even though the one going into surgery or the one who has TBI may appear calm on the outside, the reality may be that they are in shambles on the inside. Please remember, calmness is soothing. The calmer the supporters remain, the smoother the process will be for the survivor and as a whole. Supporters and survivors should try to keep the environment calm. Envision this: open the window and allow the fresh, soothing, gentle breeze to come in so that the breeze can free the reserved feelings from your body and relieve the heaviness in the air. I'm calm just imagining this.

The morning of my surgery remains vague to me. No matter how hard I try to remember the events, my recollections are few. The first thing I recall doing at the hotel was washing in the shower with the hospital's "gift" of a special blue soap, but that's all I remember about waking up and getting ready.. I recall neither the drive to the hospital nor any parts of a conversation, or if the four of us even had one. What I do recall next occurred at check-in. I remember my feeling of relief when the desk clerk said I was going to be in the Operating Room (OR) closest to the cafeteria. I was no longer concerned about Mom, Dad, and Sonia being voluntarily confined to this area. I knew in my heart that in order to remain close to me and to show their support, they wouldn't go far from me during the surgery. So my being in that particular OR made me feel closer as well.

Finally, here is the last memory I recall before my brain surgery, my lingering thought going under the anesthesia: *Medical . . . mar . . . vel, . . . heeer . . . I . . . C . . . uhhhmmmmmm . . .*

∞

Chapter 6

Awakening

At the conclusion of my four- to five-hour surgery, I was slightly awoken by the thumping heartbeat of the MRI machine. I fully awoke in the recovery room. Including all events leading up to this moment, this was a scary time for me. I was disoriented. My skull felt hot. I could also feel pressure moving outward from inside my skull. A mental picture would be of a balloon inflating, thus causing the pressure against my skull. It wasn't a balloon, though. It was my brain. I defy the idea that one's brain has no sensory stimulation because inside my brain, I could feel and hear the rhythm of my blood flowing. Pulse . . . silence . . . pulse . . . silence. This rhythm lulled me back to sleep. I was then moved to a room in the Intensive Care Unit (ICU).

The next time I awoke resembled the shining moments of the day's first rays of sunshine, the warm sun on a spring morning. It is a moment in time I will forever embrace in my heart. I opened my eyes to see my neurosurgeon, Dr. Ojemann, sitting on my good side in the room, watching me. Watching him patiently sitting there was an angel who spoke to me. The angel told me so much about what type of neurosurgeon Dr. Ojemann was and how the type of man he was made him such a wonderful, compassionate neurosurgeon. Thank you, Dr. Ojemann. I am forever grateful.

I refer to the doctor sitting on my *good* side because in addition to a massive headache, I had acquired a deep cut in my left peripheral vision. Following is a demonstration to aid you.

> *Look forward. Place your finger vertically in the center of your eye. What you can see from your finger outward, I could not. It was all black.*

Then I had my first experience of having no depth perception. Everything in the room was lined up against an invisible wall. The entire left side of my body was either very weak or wouldn't move on its own. I had to use my right arm to move my left arm or leg. The physical sensations were bizarre. They ranged from numbness to tingling throughout my body. The mental sensations were not utopian. It felt more like being in purgatory without the Christian meaning. Yes, I was physically in the room, lying in bed. However, I was experiencing an absent connection between my mind and body.

> *I could partially see and feel my body lying on the bed, but when I thought to sit up, I would continue to lie there. It was as if I were dreaming I'd gone to get a glass of water. Next came a moment of confusion upon awakening because I*

> *was still in bed with no water, my mind thinking I*
> *had gone for it, but actually I hadn't.*

Another "mind trick" happening while lying in my hospital bed was that I was observing the environment from the outside looking in, not from the inside looking out. It was a peculiar experience. The only way to describe it is "non-dimensional." To aid your understanding, an example follows.

> *Place yourself in an airplane taking a scenic*
> *flight. You are sitting by the window. When you*
> *look around, you see your body sitting in your*
> *seat . . . from outside the window! Somehow, you*
> *are physically sitting inside, while mentally, you*
> *are observing from the wing of the aircraft.*

Back to being with Dr. Ojemann. When we spoke, we briefly discussed the surgery and the immediate effects. My brain was obviously swollen from the trauma. Dr. Ojemann said an artery and motor strip had been irritated during the procedure, and it began to bleed. In time, the source had been found, then cauterized. The surgery and resections continued as planned until I began seizing. Please don't gasp. I don't believe I did. I chose to believe that my seizing at this time was a blessing.

Dr. Ojemann was mapping my brain activity, so my seizures making their "last stand" allowed him the opportunity to locate and resect the problematic areas, areas where my seizures went to hide during all the previous testing. Thankfully, he was as fiercely motivated as I. Near the end of surgery, some of the additional re-sections were located close to and in the frontal lobe and parietal region. Even though there continued to be unhealthy brain activity during surgery, Dr. Ojemann did not proceed when he came to the occipital region. I fully concur with his decisions. I have no regrets!

Others may view my seizing and additional resections as a misfortune. *Not me!* I've chosen to see them as meaning a greater probability for success, a greater probability of relief from those awful seizures! After I was updated, my response, both practical and humorous, was, "Dr. Ojemann was already in there. So hey, why not?" Only time will tell how successful the surgery was. Nevertheless, I felt comfort in knowing that I took my challenges with seizures head-on. I did everything possible not to be a victim! That is what I felt on the inside.

On the outside, with his ability to feel my slight concern and to understand my humor, he assured me that he'd left some brain for me to use. Dr. Ojemann, you have great delivery and timing for humor. I definitely needed to smile. A neurosurgeon with a sense of humor . . . I'm impressed!

In our discussion, he explained that the irritated areas had placed me in the top one percentile category for a stroke or stroke-like symptoms. I could sense the doctor's genuine concern for me. I recall my response to offer him assurance in return. "After meeting you, reviewing my tests, and after our discussions in regard to the procedures and risks," I said, "I had no reservations then, nor do I now. All will be good." Even though I was only experiencing the immediate complications at the time, unaware of the ones to follow, I still choose to believe in my own words every day . . . "All will be good."

Chapter 7
Embarkation

*T*he true outcome from recovery is unknown for an undetermined period of time. It can take months to years, depending on the "variables," the way I refer to complications. Aside from your recovery being opaque to others, the length of recovery might be one of the most frustrating challenges you will encounter. To this day, the doctors and therapists keep telling me I need to have patience. In return, I tell them, "Patience takes too long." Regardless of your personal reason or the reason of someone you know who is going to undergo brain surgery or has TBI, the mindset (no pun intended) should be that your personal discovery in your journey will take time.

Through the beginning stages of my journey, this is what I discovered about the brain. To my sister, Sonia, I remind you that I do have one. You saw the proof! I even named my brain Sally. The human brain is the most resilient, adaptable, complex, and self-defining part of an individual. My question was, "Does Sally control me, or do I control Sally?" That was pre-op.

Post-op made me realize that Sally controls me . . . to an extent. I learned that Sally is in control of my abilities, and I am in control of self-will, although these may not function harmoniously. As difficult as it was for me to do, I surrendered my trying to control her and allowed her to lead the way through my recovery. Sally and all her peers have so many things to tell, show, and teach us if we let them. Don't fight them. Embrace them! By doing so, your inner being will grow and prosper beyond what you previously "thought." I have also discovered that Stockholm syndrome does not only relate to becoming attached to your physical-hostage captor, but also to your mental-hostage captor, this being your brain during recovery. The following is an overall description of my mental-hostage captor after my brain surgery.

৪৩৪৩৪৩

I am not using text material to teach. In its place, I'm using my firsthand experiences to enlighten you. The description is to help give understanding of the resected (removed) areas and what their functions were. Next, I will describe the personal experiences the resected areas caused me to have with the immediate variables I acquired. Aside from my fascination with the procedure, giving you this information will help put occurrences in context as I continue writing. Hopefully, doing so will allow you to "see" and experience the appearance vs. reality as you continue reading.

The largest resection of my brain was the removal of my right temporal lobe. Most of a person's spatial memory and visual recognition is housed in the right temporal lobe. Two examples of how that functions are recognizing what room you're in by connecting the surrounding images to the place and knowing "who" you're looking at by connecting a face to the person, not solely to a name.

The immediate variables concerning the right temporal lobectomy were minor in the beginning. My decrease of spatial recognition introduced itself this way. In the hospital, I would leave my room for a brief time. When I returned to my room, I'd question, "Where am I? This room doesn't look familiar." I had to keep telling myself, "I'm in my room, where I'm supposed to be. I'm not lost."

The lack of visual recognition made it seem as though I was meeting the staff for the first time every time. "These professionals are not strangers," I reminded myself. "They don't mean to harm me, *even* when stabbing me with needles in my abdomen. They are supposed to be in my room." The one terrifying variable I continue to struggle with some days even now is looking in the mirror. "Is this what I look like?" I ask. I avoid mirrors whenever possible.

Therefore, after having my right temporal lobe and some of the parietal region removed, my spatial/visual *unawareness* was making the already unknown extremely difficult. It produced the intense experience of being in limbo *continuously*, followed by confusion and anxiety, along with mental and physical insecurity. My most difficult variable to cope with was the mental vulnerability I felt. People were assuring me I knew them, but I was taught growing up not to be alone with strangers or to go anywhere with them.

The second planned resection was having a portion of the hippocampus tailored. The hippocampus is where *new* incoming information is converted into long-term memories. I feel confident in saying that many memories are either in or are recalled from the hippocampus. My immediate experiences and variables concerning the hippocampus included not recalling if/what I had ordered to eat *or* if I'd even eaten. This continues today. When someone asks me what I had for dinner, I reply that I'll tell them tomorrow. In the hospital, I couldn't recall the lead nurse's name or what day of the week it was. I was continually disappointed with myself the first couple of days. I had to consistently rationalize that the recall issues were caused by all the excitement going on around me. When that didn't calm me down, I had to acknowledge that I *did* just have brain surgery. I admit that sometimes I'm a little too hard on myself and maybe expect a little too much (thus leading to disappointment and sometimes a feeling of depression).

After those first couple of days, my disappointment grew into frustration. Let me explain this transition by walking you through my experience with the lead nurse and also by describing how I interpret the cause and effects.

Following surgery, my mind became a blank slate. I went from having a full picture of a puzzle to having only a few pieces, thus the questions and answers. This was very frustrating because eventually I *did* remember that the lead nurse would ask me questions when I saw her. I *knew* the questions were coming, but I could *not* remember the answers! My personal explanation for this slow and partial recall is *repetition*. This was the opaque at work.

> *On the first day, I had no puzzle pieces to my memory recall in regard to the lead nurse. With every repetition of her coming in and doing the same thing, in the same order, I gained a half or whole piece to my puzzle. Over several days, I accumulated the recall pieces that reminded me that* first, the lead nurse would be coming in. Second, the lead nurse would ask me two questions. Third, *I remembered what the first question was.* Fourth, *I remembered what the second question was. Unfortunately, I was discharged before I acquired the pieces to the answers.*

Repetition is very important for TBI survivors and their supporters to understand and practice. I've found repetition to be a valuable recovery and coping tool, aiding integration back into daily living and helping cope with the journey into the unknown. Repetition will give you a stable grounding as the unknown becomes known again. Just remember that the more intricate the scenario, the more pieces you will have to accumulate before the puzzle is complete. I say this because I want to make sure there is no unnecessary frustration from what you may encounter. It's all right. Overall progress will vary for everyone, *but* for everyone, it will take time and repetition.

The tailored portion of the hippocampus now caused me to second-guess myself on most everything. The self-confidence I had pre-op in regard to being focused and staying on task was gone! It was an unsettling feeling. This added to my mental vulnerability. The variable created a change that stripped away a piece of who I was.

For example, how could I challenge a thought or disagree with someone if I couldn't remember what was or wasn't said?

I had to trust what unknown people were telling me. Something else I was taught early in life was to believe none of what you hear and only half of what you see. Believe only half of what I could see? Right now I could only see half of what everyone else could, literally.

As a result of this, individuals were asked to tell me when they were on my left side and to warn me if they were going to move toward me. I made this request after Sonia scared the bejeebers out of me. She didn't mean to. All she did was put something on the tray in front of me. When she did this, what I saw was an arm coming out of nowhere! Yep, I screamed.

Finally, as far as my visual deficits, the swelling caused the visualization of little gremlins or wormlike objects zipping back and forth in my lower field of vision. This was freaky. I had watched that movie! Golly geez whizzes . . . forget all I was taught growing up. Right now, I couldn't remember what I did hear or whom I met, and my visual deficits were playing tricks on me. It's not as if I couldn't make things difficult on my own. I'm very independent in that regard also!

As for the "unplanned" (during the seizing) resected pieces of my brain, they are too intricate to list and too many to name. They are scattered throughout my brain, along with areas that were either separated or disconnected from each other. When people ask me what I had done during surgery, I give the short answer. "Oh, I had a little touch-up." This reply wouldn't do justice to the reader if I had something done that you can relate to.

Following is a summary of the unplanned functions and their connections.

The majority of the unplanned areas were either linked or intertwined with my emotions on *many* levels. The connections to the limbic and central nervous system were compromised. These areas dealt with emotional responses, affective feelings, recognition of facial expressions (mad, sad, happy), ability to recognize and assess danger, and response to fear (fight or flight). The sections taken from and close to the frontal lobe also had emotional connections and functions. These pertained to my outward expressions of feelings by use of words or facial expressions. Then there were a few more resected or disconnected areas dealing with more emotions, reactions, memory recall, and cognitive processing. The resections finally ended with a little work done near the vestibular area that relates to sound/hearing and equilibrium/balance. Understand now why I say, "Oh, a little touch-up"?

You have assessed correctly if you think these unplanned areas have made an abundant contribution to the most difficult obstacles throughout my journey. They most certainly have! For one, they are opaque to the naked eye. Secondly, my terrific local neurologist, Dr. Gee, came up with a medically sophisticated phrase to summarize these emotional and cognitive variables: "It's all jazzed up in there." Even so, I still have no regrets about the surgery. I remain thankful I seized when I did.

As a coping skill, I just have to put my practice of repetition into use. When I break down in tears or become discombobulated, I say, "I'm very sorry. It's not you. It's my inability to regulate my emotional response." This is the medically sophisticated way Dr. Cossaboon, my fabulous neuropsychologist, explained my emotional meltdowns. For the first six months of recovery, I kept a note with me at all times with these words written down. Sounds silly, but it worked and proved useful. Don't hesitate to do the same if you need to.

As I stated before, no two recoveries are identical or have the same variables. In my recovery, I have also learned that these variables will present themselves at various times over the course of recovery. Keeping the description of my brain surgery and immediate variables in mind . . . you are now beginning the journey into my self-discovery.

Chapter 8

Self-Discovery

*T*he remainder of my post-op, I was engrossed with self-discovery. "Self-discovery" is how I define me, the patient/survivor, learning the existence of my unknown difficulties in real time. These difficulties were continuously creating "Post-Op Sandra." Looking back, I strongly wish we (my supporters and I) had had prior awareness, along with the mind-set of a new beginning, before the surgery. If we'd had these, I deeply believe that much of the frustration and disappointment that followed would have been avoided.

I would like our mishaps to be noticed, but my only intention in sharing is to help others achieve a more successful, productive, less frustrating, and less stressful recovery. There are absolutely no hard feelings on my behalf toward anyone. All is good, my loved ones and friends. I definitely contributed my fair portion to the frustration throughout our journey in recovery (and life in general).

In hindsight, as a whole, we should have taken away

the assumptions of Pre-Op Sandra concerning my mental and physical functions and abilities. We should have begun this new era with a clean slate and an open mind. Out with the old (Pre-Op) Sandra and in with the new (Post-Op) Sandra. Oh, but not my personality traits, thank goodness. They have remained intact. I'm still trying to figure out what Dr. Ojemann meant in his reply to me after surgery. I was obsessing in the Neuro Acute Care Unit (NACU) about being able to begin graduate school in the upcoming summer, and he said, "Oh. You're one of those." Hmm? Guess I'll take it as a compliment. Thank you, Doctor.

I encourage anyone in this situation and anyone who has acquired other forms of TBI to start anew. Make it easier on yourself. You might have enough to work through with just the basics. Don't make it more difficult for yourself by holding to the notion that nothing will change, because it *will*. The changes that occur will be at different levels for everyone, but the changes *will* be there.

My advice to patients is to keep an open mind, to hold no expectations of yourself or others, and to stay strong with a positive attitude. This is a new beginning where you can use your previous life lessons, wisdom, and maturity to manage your growth. Unfortunately, at least for me, we didn't have some of these values during our growth period through adolescence. Nevertheless, for most of us now, we do. That alone is a huge positive!

My advice to the supporters is also to hold no expectations of anyone. Before reacting, keep in the forefront of your thoughts what the patient has just undergone. Accept that there will be differences in the patient for a time. It's understandable to not want a loved one to have difficulties, but just accept it with openness. Choose to make post-op your "patient-discovery" time. You can do so by asking the professionals questions, if you have any. "What can I/we do to help relieve the patient's anxiety?" is a valuable question. Continue your discovery by asking the patient questions slowly! "Can you . . .? Do you feel up to . . .?" And most importantly, "Are you able to . . .?" They might not know yet themselves, but please don't assume *anything!*

I'm not sure how to proceed in regard to my stay/ incarceration in the hospital. (That's a joke—I think.) Many things were taking place. The second morning after surgery, I was moved from the Intensive Care Unit to the Neuro Acute Care Unit. The staff was great at immediately getting me up and moving. Also, there were several doctors, interns, a physical therapist (PT), an occupational therapist (OT), and a speech and language pathologist (SLP) coming in and out of my room to administer evaluations.

Keeping my brain surgery and variables in mind, I realize I was becoming discombobulated from the visual movements surrounding me, trying to process directions during the evaluations, and being in an unfamiliar environment. Of course my head was still swollen. It felt hot inside and throbbed with pain. The visual deficits in my left eye were tripping me out. My physical inability to move normally was very frightening. Lastly, I was so tired.

Any amount of physical *or* mental exertion caused uncontrollable fatigue. For example, after walking the twenty feet (using my walker) to my bathroom and back,

I would return to the bed and immediately fall into a deep sleep. The same goes for the PT and OT evaluations. Whether they took place outside my room or on my bed, it didn't matter. I would be in a deep sleep afterward. When the SLP came in to administer his evaluation, after several minutes I began drifting off on him. Oops, my bad. Hope you didn't take it personally.

Summing up these few experiences in an analogy, I'd say they produced a sensation resembling the sound and movement of the swirling wind in a tornado, combined with the intense pounding and pressure of a hurricane, simultaneously taking place in my little skull. It encouraged me to want to curl up in a little ball to sleep and dream the pain and confusion away.

The outcome was only empty sleep as an escape. In my case, I did not dream for almost a year after brain surgery. I was happy about not dreaming due to my history of nocturnal seizures. Remember, previously my dreams were my déjà vu precursor before seizing. This followed by being awoken by a vile smell that made me feel nauseated and physically sick. Therefore, no dreaming was a happy slumber!

ಙಀಙಀಙ

While I was trying to adapt and function successfully with this sensation of a storm in my skull, my loving family was trying their best to comfort me. This leads me to why I wish we all had had prior awareness and an open mind to our own discoveries and had held no assumptions or expectations after my surgery. Also, this is why it is so important to start anew! Sometimes the comforting without this mind-set caused added frustration.

The feelings I encountered in the hospital were nobody's fault and not to be taken personally. We all did our best. We meant well for each other. For instance, the first or second day out of ICU, my thoughtful father called my aunt from my room to give her an update. That was fine. Spontaneously handing me the phone to say hello and to talk . . . was not. Pre-Op Sandra would have had no problem taking the phone to say hello. Post-Op Sandra did!

My first reaction to having the phone handed to me without warning was being startled. The spontaneity of the action caused visual and mental confusion. What came next was anxiety. While my mind was already jumbled, I was trying to place who my aunt was (memory recall). Then I felt frustration because my spoken words were slow and what was coming out wasn't the same as what I was thinking (acquired aphasia). In the end, I became angry and disappointed in myself for not being able to hold a conversation or answer random questions (delay in cognitive processing). These feelings I encountered from learning the existence of the unknown in my self-discovery manifested in anger!

My anger was hard to contain and control. This led me to outwardly express my inner anxiety, frustration, and disappointment in myself. I abruptly handed the phone back to Dad without saying good-bye. Sorry, Aunt Kathy. Our first confrontation with the unknown caused a little riff in the room. We all became frustrated with ourselves, with each other, and mostly with the unknown.

"What is happening?" became the prevailing indirect question in the room. "Why are you acting like that?"

was the supporters' offensive question to me. *"Can't you see* I'm recovering from TBI?" was my irritated unspoken question to all of them present. The answer to my question was no! Remember, TBI is opaque. It is difficult for others to know what the patient is going through because it's not visible. Hence, I'm sharing to help all of you be aware of and to understand what is happening or to prepare for what might happen.

After reading about this event, some could conclude that I had, and have, hard feelings toward others. In actuality, it's just the opposite. The phone experience makes a great example regarding two critical needs people *must* understand. The first is why everyone needs the post-op mind-set of self-discovery, patient-discovery, no expectations or assumptions, having an open mind concerning the patient's functions and abilities, acknowledging and taking into consideration what the patient has just undergone, and starting anew. The second is the *imperative* need for everyone to meet with a neuropsychologist. Either meet before the procedure or as soon as possible after *any* TBI.

Wow, Dad! All of this was learned by you handing me the phone. It wasn't a pleasant experience at the time for any of us, although now it will help many people preparing for their discovery and recovery. You are assisting in helping beyond me in an enduring way. You are the world's best, Dad!

ೞೞೞ

In addition to this surrounding chaos, having the wide spectrum of staff and others in my room was also mentally overwhelming and tiring. Having lived alone for a long period of time did not help me with this particular adjustment. I was accustomed to personal space and quiet time to reflect and plan ahead. Being confined in the hospital didn't help. I felt like such a burden to my family. My family also enjoys being active and visiting new places. With my incarceration, I felt as if I was taking away from their time—time they could spend doing fun stuff and being adventurous. As a solution to all, I encouraged Dad, Mom, and Sonia to at least go down to the market. It took a lot of persuading, but they eventually gave in and went.

While they were away, I used my alone time wisely, that is, in between staff visits and drifting off to sleep. I needed this time to try to evaluate my situation and to plan accordingly. My first objective was to find out how I could get out of there. Rehabilitation Medicine felt I would benefit from a stay in the Inpatient Rehab. While in Inpatient Rehab, I would receive daily intensive therapies. The proposed time period would begin after my surgical recovery. Even though I concurred with their assessments, I longed to return home . . . to reunite with my "physical constant."

My personal belief is that most individuals have two "constants" in their life, the first being a "spiritual constant," the second being a "physical constant." These are my personal definitions of the two constants.

> *By spiritual constant, I mean a person's choice of a higher power or being if they choose to have one. A spiritual constant contributes to your inner strength and provides comfort. This constant is intangible but is always with you. It's not based on what faith you practice or even if you practice*

a faith. As long as your choice of a higher power or being is loving, non-harmful to yourself or to others, and also brings a positive and comforting feeling, then all is good.

By physical constant, I mean someone or something that is familiar to you and is tangible. It gives you security and comfort in a physical form (nonsexual). It's a consistent grounding when one is confused, stressed, panicked, insecure, or vulnerable. Someone or something you can depend on to be there for you during these events, a safety net, per se. Some individuals have a spouse, friend, or pet as their physical constant. The physical constant welcomes you and enwraps you in a sense of safety and familiarity with no visible changes. It's reliable.

I share openly who and what my constants are. My spiritual constant is my Lord Jesus Christ. He is always in my heart and never makes me feel alone. I can depend on him to be available at all times. My God helps guide me when I'm lost and comforts me internally when I'm scared. When I have concerns, he aids me in finding the positive, therefore becoming my spiritual constant. He was with me in the hospital.

In this era of my life, my only physical constant was my home. Don't feel pity for me, because I sure don't. Here are the reasons for my home being my physical constant. My dearest friends and family lived a great distance from me. I chose to not have a pet until I could sustain my own health and responsibilities. Over the past couple of years, my illness had built a barrier between myself and having a close personal relationship.

The last reason is that my stubborn independence caused me to alienate myself from all others without realizing it. These reasons made my home my physical constant. This is where I would retreat when I felt sick, confused, scared, and insecure in my surroundings. I would consistently feel safe and protected when at home.

ঙঙঙ

Lying in my hospital bed, I tried to remain focused. My thoughts were scattered, though. I kept repeating, "How can I make this happen? How can I reunite with my physical constant?" I felt it would be more beneficial to my recovery to be home . . . to feel secure with familiarity around me, to consistently wake up and recognize where I was, to be in a known place, to have the ability to control my surroundings, and to have grounding. This included my visual and auditory intake. I needed to return home to feel complete and secure. *What do I need to do to make this happen? Think, Sandra . . . Make a checklist!*

My parents were already planning to return home with me. They were willing to stay as long as needed. Great! Having live-in help arranged . . . I could check that off my needs-to-return-home list. Now, what about my therapies? Oh duh, Post-Op Sandra!

At the time, I worked for an excellent nonprofit organization, which is dedicated to early detection and intervention for children. My coworkers and friends were a mix of SLPs, OTs, and PTs. Plus, my boss, Mitch, my guardian angel, reassured me before I left that he would do whatever it took to help me post-op. Mitch, who understood me, made me promise to ask him or my coworkers if I needed anything.

Therefore, my internal debate began.

> Sandra, ask for help with your therapies.
> *Huh? Ask for help?*
> Yes, Sandra.
> *Concede I'm not Superwoman or a medical marvel—YET!*
> **YES,** Sandra.
> *GIVE UP SOME OF MY INDEPENDENCE?*
> **YES**, SANDRA!
> *BURDEN OTHERS WITH MY PROBLEMS?*
> **YOU'RE NOT! THEY'RE YOUR FRIENDS! DO IT NOW!**

This was too much for me. Nevertheless, after my internal debate, I took a big gulp of pride and a baby step. I decided to contact the first person who came into my thoughts. Hmm? Oh, Nancy!

Please allow me to expand for a moment beyond my lessons learned during recovery. I want to share a lesson learned from my life. It's also an inspirational event. The valuable life lesson is to offer an olive branch. This gesture is an opening into something profound and endearing. Without exaggeration, for me it was life-altering.

The lesson goes as follows. When I began working with my friends/therapists as an SLP assistant, Nancy supervised me. In addition to viewing Nancy as my supervisor, I saw her as my professional mentor. I've always looked up to her. She is an amazing speech therapist with a very kind soul! Nancy also instills the commitment and passion to help others. Unfortunately, at this time there was an underlying tension between us. Please don't misunderstand me and misinterpret what I'm writing. The tension between Nancy and me was not personally directed toward or from either of us It was just there.

I couldn't figure out the reason for this tension. Being a new employee, I was too worried to make waves by pursuing the issue. Instead, I just went with it. I learned as much as I could about my profession as an upcoming SLP, and I did what I was asked to do. Even though the tension bothered me, I wanted so much to impress Nancy and to earn her respect. I knew I could never measure up to be her equal as an SLP, but I wanted to come as close as I could. I did not want to disappoint Nancy with my job performance nor let her down personally. This led to another self-debate.

> Sandra, reach out to Nancy.
> *Will my contacting her add to the tension?*
> Sandra, you won't know if you don't TRY.
> *Will my current difficulties disappoint her?*
> Do you really believe that?
> *Okay, self, what would Nancy do in my situation?*
> Good question. Nancy is also tenacious with a take-charge attitude!

In conclusion, I made the call to Nancy and asked for her help with my need for cognitive therapy. By doing so, I offered an olive branch. Thankfully, Nancy accepted. Not only did she respond with a simple yes, she sounded excited to help with an open heart and gave me assurance. At this time I was unaware the assurance wasn't confined to just my therapies. It continues to blossom, thus becoming life-altering.

Nancy has become a personal mentor, an advocate, a confidant, and a human constant throughout my recovery, a strong, steady pillar for me to lean on when my emotions become unsteady. Since our reunion when I returned home, Nancy has been very tuned in to my mental and physical cues. When I'm nearing the cliff of emotional instability, she is quick to be beside me so that I don't fall into the abyss of spiraling emotions.

For example, Nancy and I were seated at a table with three others. As a group, we were trying to have an important discussion. I was becoming mentally overwhelmed, along with being visually and auditorily overstimulated. First, I began to physically shake. Then my lip began to quiver, followed by tears.

Just as I was about to fall into the abyss, Nancy got up, walked around the table, and knelt beside me. She proceeded to lightly rub my arm while reassuring me that I was doing well and among friends. Thanks to her keen senses and kindness, I calmed down, or as I now say, "leveled out," much sooner than I would have without her.

Afterward, I thanked her profusely. What she said in return meant more than words. Nancy graciously replied, "No need to thank me. I could feel you hurting." You're right, Nancy. I don't need to thank you. I need to thank my God for having you in my life. I do so every day!

Most importantly, along with becoming a dear friend, Nancy has become my compass when I can very easily veer off course. She does everything from helping me to prioritize my daily, weekly, and monthly goals to making sure I don't get confused and wander off in the grocery store. Also, when buying groceries, she makes sure I stick to my list! That's an accomplishment for anyone to achieve with me.

Nancy has contributed to my feeling of being blessed. Thank you so much! You are truly appreciated by me and my family. I continue to look up to you every day. No pressure, my dear friend.

I hope this event will inspire others to extend an olive branch in your time of need. Please don't hesitate to offer peace to those you admire. In my doing so, I can say with joy, "Peace and Nancy are priceless."

Returning back to my hospital room, I could now check SLP off my needs-to-return-home list. The next thing I did was to reach out to two other coworkers and dear friends, Kim and Sharon. They, too, are wonderful therapists and confidants. Kim and Sharon graciously agreed, also without hesitation and with open hearts, to help me so I could return home. I was very much looking forward to seeing them and hopefully having a good laugh about something other than me. *Ah, relief. Therapies are taken care of.*

With Nancy, Kim, and Sharon helping me during my recovery, I became blessed with having the greatest support team known to man! They are fantastic role models and references for what it takes to become an exceptional support team. They each have a special gift for helping. I am so blessed to be the recipient. Hopefully, my sharing with you will be accepted as my way of paying it forward.

After contacting everyone, I developed a strong case for returning home. The doctors were impressed with my resources, but they were being very cautious about discharging me. They insisted that I wait a few more days. This was not because they wanted to increase my bill. They wanted to make certain I had the ability to strengthen my physical weakness and to become self-sufficient while remaining safe. That's another good value to have in your doctors. With their justifiable reasoning, I lay back in my bed and tried to be a good patient *with* "patience."

During the waiting period for me to be well enough for discharge, my family and I kept ourselves occupied and entertained, sometimes at my expense. To anyone with siblings, visualize this: there I was in my room, sitting up in bed with a huge cone of gauze around my head, in *pain* until the nurse or doctor started the morphine drip. Now, even though I was unable to play Scrabble with Sonia, she found a way to stay entertained. What did Sonia do? My dear sister whipped out her cell phone, began taking pictures of me, then forwarded them to family and friends! Siblings out there, can you feel my "pain"? It was all good. We laughed. She more than I, but we laughed.

From Sonia's sisterly eagerness to share the pictures, I recall two replies. The first came from Deb, the second exchange sister my family hosted when I was in high school. She and I have maintained very strong sisterly bonds over the years, along with a strong family bond as a whole. Deb's reply to Sonia was "Ohhh, Sandra should be so happy to know her picture is now seen throughout Europe!"

"*Oh*, sisters!" I responded.

The next reply came from Nancy. She said she couldn't believe I was smiling.

"I met my new friend . . . *morphine!*" I told her.

Sonia might have felt a little bad sending the pictures, although—I say this with sisterly love—I doubt it. Anyway, she gave me the cutest and softest little teddy bear from my five-year-old nephew, Tyler. I felt touched. Tyler is a very special piece in my puzzle of life. I always refer to him as my chicken soup, meaning the comfort for my soul. I loved the bear. The nurses put a duplicate of my ID band on the bear's wrist. Tyler would be happy to know that the bear remains seated on top of my dresser at home to watch over me at night. Thank you, Tyler. Okay, sis, even trade-off for the humiliation! Nice save on your side.

The "sisterly fun" increased after the gauze was removed. My long, naturally curly hair was matted from being wrapped for days with the sweat, blood, and antiseptic gel on my scalp. We couldn't get a comb to move through it. I wasn't allowed to wash my scalp for several more days. This created a double-edged sword. My scalp itched terribly, but if I touched it to try and relieve the itch, it caused pain. Sonia's suggestion? "Let's cut the mats out!" Translation? "Ohhh, my pretty. How I've wanted to cut off your curly hair since we were little. Now I can without getting in trouble!" (Are you picturing the green lady with the wart on her nose?)

I'll give Sonia credit for first trying to find someone in the hospital to cut it, then someone to help her with cutting it. There was no one to help. I was a little hesitant, *but* Sonia was kind enough to take more pictures to show me how bad it looked. She shared those also!

On a serious side note, for any hairstylist who would like to volunteer their time, this would be a thoughtful and useful way to extend your services. Ask your local hospital if they will allow you to assist in making a patient's stay more comfortable. I'm not making this suggestion from vanity, only from sincerity.

That said, Sonia made her point. Along with feeling uncomfortable, my look was bad. I appeared to have oversized dreadlocks coated with blood and the antiseptic gel. My surgical wound was a big C carved in the right side of my head. (I said the C stood for cute, but nobody was buying it.) In the center of the C was a long, thin braid of hair the surgeons used to pull my scalp back. Glad I could help you, gentlemen. Therefore, my response to Sonia was, "Sure. Have at it." Was this trust or vulnerability? Just kidding, sis. I trusted you and enjoyed it almost as much as you did . . . well, maybe.

When Sonia finished with gusto, there appeared to be a furry little dog sitting on my lap. At least I looked a little younger. I went from being matty to natty. How do I know this? *Yep* . . . Sonia took more pictures! I did appreciate the haircut, though. My scalp was very sensitive to pain when touched. The matted and encrusted hair also caused hurt when touched or moved. My "new style" offered some relief from the itching, so it felt great to get rid of the mats.

What didn't feel so good, though, came after the haircutting ceremony.

Dad, Mom, and Sonia took another trip to the market. They were thinking of me and what might cheer me up. Sonia picked out and brought back something from a bakery that looked wonderful and smelled delicious. How yummy and thoughtful! Something other than Cream of Wheat to eat. I opened my jaw for a mouthwatering, savory bite when suddenly I experienced a sharp, stabbing pain that caused me to lose my breath.

The pain shot up from the right side of my jaw to my right temple. Another self-discovery, I was only able to open my jaw from maybe a quarter to a half inch. This pain was caused from the surgical procedures of having to cut and suture the temporalis muscle, dislocate and relocate the temporomandibular joint (I'm using the surgeon's verbiage), and from the residual swelling.

Needless to say, I wasn't able to eat the bakery morsel because I could barely open my mouth. I believe my dear sister's comment in regard to my decreased mandibular mobility went something like this: "Hey, you should have had this surgery long ago!" Oh well, it's the thought that matters.

After a total of five full days in the hospital, on the morning of the sixth day, I was released from my incarceration.

ℬ

Chapter 9

Entering the Threshold

*T*he day before my release, Sonia returned to Denver. Without her, my mental and physical entrapment heightened. I no longer had an inner escape. My comic relief was no longer next to me. This void increased my eagerness to leave the confinement of the hospital, so when the doctors signed for my discharge, I felt freedom approaching, only to have it quickly swept aside.

While preparing to leave, my mind began swirling with confusion, frustration, and anxiety. Also, the slight pressure I felt by being rushed, though not by the staff, to make discharge time made everything mentally overwhelming. We were all eager to leave, but please remember, there needs to be a blanket of calmness.

This is a summary of the immediate struggle I was trying to overcome in making my discharge time.

I *cognitively* knew what I had to do before leaving, such as change clothes, sign papers, and pack. Oh, I couldn't forget Sally (my brain)! It just wasn't happening. There was an unseen disconnect between identifying and executing a task. I was "lost in transition." My mental *thoughts* were running randomly like a herd of wild horses fleeing from the corral, while my *thought process* and *physical actions* were moving lethargically, resembling a pack of mules going up a mountain! Eventually, I got the "giddy" in my "up." I was leaving the hospital!

My last action as a hospital (not-so-patient) patient was to sit in a wheelchair, waiting to be taken downstairs. In hindsight, Sally and I were unprepared for what lay ahead. "We" had no forewarning as to what could be waiting for us on the other side of the doors. When being wheeled through the exit, to our unknowing, Sally and I were entering the threshold of the unknown frontier. Dad, Mom, Sally, and I climbed into a taxi and rode off to the hotel.

Unfortunately, nothing in TBI recovery is simple. Please don't let this discourage you. I promise there is always a positive during the difficult times—that is, if you *choose* to acknowledge and accept it. My mind-set in life has been that "knowledge is power." This means I've chosen to learn from personal experiences to empower myself. I refuse to allow brain surgery to alter this particular mind-set of mine. Therefore, my outlook embarking on my journey into the unknown frontier became: "The more I experience, the more I can learn to empower myself." I aspire to empower you also by sharing with you what I have learned thus far during recovery.

After leaving the hospital, what came next were my "first steps." Getting out of the taxi was my first attempt using the walker on unfamiliar ground. It was a physical struggle. I needed assistance so I wouldn't fall down or tip over. With my physical weakness, visual deficits, lack of coordination, and imbalance, I was *not* as proficient with the walker as I'd been striving for. After making it inside our hotel suite, I slept for a bit. I slept to take a physical rest and a mental break from all the challenges and variables Sally and I were encountering. Unfortunately, it was a short break.

Once I'd awoken, new challenges and variables awaited. They were much more eager to present themselves to Sally and me than we were to meet them! A mental picture I have for this moment of "awakening" is this:

> *An anxious mob of challenges and variables waited outside my bedroom door. Some were fighting each other to get to me first. Others were lingering in the back, waiting for their right moment to come forward. The remainder of challenges and variables were above, like vultures, circling around with their beady little eyes fixed on me. They were waiting for the perfect time to strike, to strike when their "prey" was off guard. Although each carried a different mission to mayhem, their goal was the same ... to be the strongest and to last the longest.*

If only the mass mob would have been courteous enough to form a line, thus allowing Sally and me to meet each individually, then sparing us time to learn how to cope with one before moving on to meet the next. If the challenges and variables had been merciful, the outcome to date might have been in our favor. *But noooo!* That wasn't in their "challenges and variables playbook."

They made a mistake, though. They had the playbook for a "common" game. Well, guess what, challenges and variables? This is *not* a common game. I have been told repeatedly in life that I am *not* a common person. (I choose to accept that as a compliment.) I am beginning my journey through the unknown frontier. I am committed to surviving, holding my ground, and moving forward, and I'm too proud to surrender! This is *not* a game. This is *war!*

Now that I have that off my chest, let's continue in the hotel suite.

The events that followed continue the patient- and self-discovery. The immediate challenges and variables we confronted were numerous. They mirrored the additional resected areas of my brain, in that they were many and intricate. Even so, I will now begin to list and describe each as they occurred. My variables in the hospital continued to exist. In addition to or originating from those, these were my new variables and self-discoveries that no one could see.

Auditory overstimulation (AO) was caused by all sounds (stimuli). This ranged from the television being on to the noise of making meals in the kitchen. The slightest auditory stimuli would startle me/Sally and was amplified. The amplification was due to the fluid buildup in the right ear. Sometimes the increased volume brought tears to my eyes.

Along with the increased amount of stimuli I could hear, I also became confused by each individual sound. If anyone who was unaware of my current situation saw my physical reaction, he or she might have thought I was only experiencing a bad headache. This is what couldn't be seen:

> *The confusion took place when Sally was trying first to identify the sound (cognitive recognition), and second to connect the sound to the origin of what was making it (cognitive processing with memory recall). This delay was followed by trying to process how I should react (limbic and central nervous system). Fight or flight?*
>
> *For example, Mom took a pot out of the cabinet and a lid fell. Sally took the AO bang and tried to identify what made it, then where it came from. Let's think . . . did a door close inside or on a car outside? Did someone fall inside? Was somebody outside hitting on our door? The final reaction to the AO was "Am I safe?"*

The new variable was very confusing and frightening. At this moment I discovered that my auditory processing was delayed from my cognition. Additionally, I subconsciously discovered the significance of the compromised connections going to and from my brain, limbic, and central nervous system (CNS) after the surgery. *Oh my goodness, Sandra! If a stranger broke in, would I be able to cognitively process and react fast enough to save myself or others?*

Visual overstimulation (VO) took place when I became overstimulated by visual objects (stimuli). Whether the objects were stationary or moving, they confused me and increased my anxiety. The mass portion of my resections in the right temporal lobe and some of my parietal region was the prominent cause for Sally and my VO.

These resected areas affected the relationship to most stationary objects and spaces in my surrounding environment. Some of the smaller resections and their locations were also to blame. They increased VO caused by movements. Let me break it down for you in my own words, using my own experiences.

My object, facial, and spatial recognition (visual identification) was still compromised, just as it had been in the hospital. When you have an uncompromised brain, after you walk into a room, you know where you are physically (kinesthetic awareness). It's also a natural instinct when you see someone you know (visual recognition), to react with pleasantries. After the surgery, fewer things came naturally to me.

My natural reaction to seeing people I'd known changed. Yes, I mean to use past tense. Pre-Op Sandra would see someone she'd recognize and say, "Hello! How are you?" Post-Op Sandra now saw someone and was mystified. *Who is that?* I would think. *Do I know, or should I know?* The answers to these questions were previously clarified by the right temporal lobe (which I no longer had), the parietal region, and the hippocampus (which I now had less of).

The right temporal lobe and parietal region also stored my visual and spatial memories (surrounding environment). My immediate visual/spatial variable expanded outside the perimeter of the hospital. It pursued me vigorously after my discharge and continues to this day! For this reason, my challenge with being aware/unaware of my visual/spatial surroundings merits its own term, "Sandra's spatial oblivion."

My spatial oblivion/unawareness has caused me to

question every place I go. Attaching itself to my oblivion are self-doubt, insecurity, and vulnerability. The unforeseen experience is surreal in an unpleasant way. It alone has given me three personal challenges: to understand *what* I am experiencing in real time, to articulate the experience, and to discover what determines kinesthetic awareness or unawareness. After eighteen months of personal research, I'm optimistic about helping TBI survivors (who share my oblivion) understand what they're experiencing and why.

During my stay in the hospital, I was introduced to the unawareness. The introduction took place going to/from the bathroom and in/out of my room. The intro was minor compared to the broader experiences in the hotel suite. The broadness of my oblivion seemed to equal the broadness of the spatial environment. Our suite was a small apartment in comparison to my hospital room. Therefore, after discharge, I was venturing deeper into my spatial oblivion.

A couple of nights into our stay at the suite, I thought I was comfortable and familiar being in this new environment, but when going into the living room to sit down, I was unknowingly walking deeper into Sandra's oblivion. Let me welcome you into my unwelcome experience.

> I sat down on the couch and began to feel uneasy. It was the same feeling you may experience before something bad happens or when you're walking through a dark alley and you have an unexplained impulse to keep looking behind you. Also, you may have an inexplicable urge to run!

This is the unpleasant, surreal feeling I referred to earlier. So sitting on the couch, I looked around the room. To see if everything was all right? To see if I could identify what was making me feel this way?

What I saw were objects that had no identity to me. I knew I saw a chair, but whose chair was it? I don't know who this chair belongs to, so whose room am I in? *I thought. In my oblivion, I felt ungrounded and detached from my surrounding environment.*

While this experience was taking place in the room, this is what was taking place in my mind. Readers, think of this mental process as that of a good journalist confirming before believing by coordinating details. Here is my thought process.

Have I been here before? *The answers I received from memory recall were incomplete. Sally's ability to recall my being somewhere physically had been preserved. Therefore, Sally could answer that I had physically been here. My mental unawareness emerged when I couldn't recall anything else. I was unable to recall details to* confirm *Sally's answer that I was here before. Why?*

The answer I'm sharing isn't based on professional medical findings. I'm using my own layman's words from my personal research. I believe the origin of my spatial oblivion took place during surgery, when the majority of my stored spatial details vanished with their correlating areas. For writing purposes, I've named all memory recall areas for spatial and visual awareness Bob. The few remnants of details that Bob kept (remained intact) caused ambiguity.

Using my thought process from above with the new knowledge of Bob, I will explain the *why*. When Sally was able to recall, "Yes, you've been here," Bob was unable to continue the thought process by recalling details. "I don't recall anything that looks familiar. Are you sure?" was his reply. In the end, I was unable to confirm what I was thinking. Therefore, I couldn't believe where I was with any confidence.

The inability to recall details cast continuous self-doubt. Its impact caused insecurity, anxiety, and panic. Staying with the same thought process, I will describe the emotional process that took place simultaneously, my newly discovered apprehension and the kinesthetic unawareness I felt. This was my *personal experience*.

> "Have I been here before?" I asked.
> Sally answered, "Yes, you've physically been here before."
> I felt calm and secure. Then I turned to Bob to recall details to confirm, to find familiarity and truth.
> Bob answered, "I don't recall any details."
> That ended the experience with personal feelings of insecurity, panic, and self-doubt.

My personal thoughts during these types of experiences . . . I didn't *know* anything with only one exception, I now knew the feeling of "being lost." Wherever I went, I felt lost. I was desperate to return home to my physical constant, to feel safe and grounded. Oh, and readers, don't worry about Sally and Bob answering me. They're only a metaphor. I am being treated for TBI, not schizophrenia!

For TBI survivors, if you have this *bizarre* experience, remember that you're not crazy, either! A simple way to determine if you are experiencing unawareness or just having an "off" day is this: A-ble to recall details equals A-wareness. UN-able to recall details equals UN-awareness.

Supporters, you can help survivors through this emotional experience by talking with them, not solely in common dialogue, but by reminiscing about items in the environment. From my experience, I strongly recommend this approach. Reintroduce the environment from what you, the supporters, remember, not from the position of what the survivor doesn't recall. "I had such fun when we shopped for your couch!"

Supporters, by implementing this approach, you will help survivors become more aware in a calm, casual, productive way. In addition, it takes the survivors' focus away from the unaware that may cause them panic, insecurity, self-doubt, and occasionally the inability to regulate their emotional responses. You are redirecting away from the survivors' unawareness to the supporters' awareness.

Soon after my discovery of VO and kinesthetic unawareness, a new visual variable and challenge came forward . . . Sally wasn't in sync with my eyes. This occurred with people and most moving objects. The source might have been the resected areas going back toward the occipital lobe. Regardless of its origin, this optical disconnect caused me to visualize movements that I can only compare to either an action book or cartoon illustrations, courtesy of Sally.

Sally's inspiration for the action-book illustrations resulted from her trying to function efficiently. During my surgery, various pages (brain) had been removed. Also, some pathways to retrieve images were no longer connected. New pathways had to be rebuilt. Because rebuilding takes recovery time, Sally had to skip sequential movements to keep up with the incoming visual stimuli. Hence, Sally created what I call "the action-book effect." This was her illustration through my eyes.

> When I saw someone walking or other types of actions, I would see nothing but their partial movements. The unseen or "skipped" portions resembled flipping through an older action book, one that had an action sequence drawn on each page. In my case, some of the pages were missing. So when Sally flipped the pages quickly (trying to process the incoming visual stimuli as fast as it was received), the objects appeared to skip sequences in their movements.

To help you understand this experience, imagine the following. You see someone standing or moving on your right. You blink your eyes. The person is now standing or moving on your left. This was my experience. Only, I never blinked. It was just a missing page.

In due time, Sally was able to try processing some visual movements. When she did, she compensated for the skipped images by using "fillers." This created the "cartoon effect." "Sally's trying her hardest to function correctly," I would repeat to myself, as a way of rationalizing what I was experiencing visually. It kept me sane when seeing such things as:

> *Some objects were being followed by a long, dark shadow or an elongated image of the object. Have you ever seen a person five feet tall and seven feet long when they walk by? Now a dinner plate. Have you ever seen it transform its shape right in front of you?*

To aid you in this experience, imagine you are looking down at your plate. Somebody slides it over to one side, and it expands from a round plate into an oval platter. To me these images resembled what you'd see when cartoon characters run on television. Ah . . . television. After explaining the images, all I need to say is that, "These examples were multiplied by however many actions there were on the screen."

Along with my vision deficits, I began to experience vertigo caused by the fluid in my right ear. I became nauseated from the sensation of intense spinning. When my eyes were open, the spinning reminded me of the tight air spins we did when I jumped tandem at thirteen-thousand feet. It was definitely the opposite feeling of the encompassing serenity I experienced when doing the world's highest parasailing on a calm, sunny day. Guess those fun days are over . . . killjoy. When I would lie down and close my eyes, I had to keep one foot on the floor, just like the college days, to stop the room from spinning . . . *Uhhh*, so I heard, Mom. (No killjoy here!)

Finally, about the vertigo, it obviously worsened my

balance. For me to stand vertically without my walker was not safe. To sit in an armless chair was just as challenging. Whenever my torso was vertical and I was stationary, I'd catch myself swaying. The lack of balance definitely made it difficult to be outside on a windy Wyoming day!

The physical weakness I had experienced in the hospital became prevalent. The more I tried to function, the more strenuous simple functions became. I was too weak to lift an empty dinner plate. I couldn't raise a small glass any longer than to take a sip. I had to rest my arm several times when brushing my teeth. Lastly, I didn't have the strength to open and close a snap or button.

Every example occurred when using both hands, which I began to do consistently because I couldn't keep from shaking. I believe my shaking was due to muscle weakness, "elephant strength" medications, and anxiety. Also, Mom continues to remind me that I would eat very little. I vaguely remember something about her saying that I could eat it myself, or she could make me. I'm joking, I think.

My coordination was almost extinct. It took great effort to connect a zipper, place my foot in a shoe, or put on a coat. It was also difficult to rub moisture cream on my face. Seriously. *If* I was strong enough to open the jar of face cream *and* made contact with my face, I would apply it either in my ear or in my eye. Not to mention, it tasted horrible! Yes, I was looking in the mirror. Having no depth perception while looking in the mirror was only half the problem. I'll get to the other half later.

Something I *was* successful at was becoming physically fatigued, same as in the hospital. Only now, it increased from walking several feet into tiring after daily tasks—tasks such as brushing my teeth, getting dressed, and eating! Completing these physical tasks resulted in continuous naps. After I thought I could cope with the physical fatigue, the mental/cognitive fatigue began. My variables were relentless! This was my next self-discovery.

When I attempted to watch five minutes of television, I was met by the additional challenge of trying to cognitively *follow* what was being said, not solely the spoken words, but also their meaning. Recall that I had lost parts of Sally that enabled me to understand non-literal meanings and innuendoes and to identify facial expressions, along with emotional or affective feelings. Therefore, whatever I heard from a person's mouth was processed as *literal* meaning.

These are my thoughts when trying to follow the dialog:

"Man, what's your problem?" *Why aren't you answering him? What IS your problem? Did I miss something? . . .* Confusion.

"Hey, you want to come back to my place, baby?" *Why? Do you know her? Did I miss something? . . .* Confusion.

At the same time, I was trying to cognitively *identify* the nonverbal. Whatever expression I saw on a person's face had *no* meaning.

The actor asked, "Do I look mad?" *Well, I personally don't know. . . .* Confusion. *What does mad look like? . . .* Confusion. *Someone please tell me! Ugh . . .* More confusion!

Needless to say, that time was very frustrating. I had to concede that Sally and I weren't ready for television. It was not mentally possible. To summarize my experience trying to watch TV having AO, VO, and the inability to identify and process verbal and non-verbal meanings . . . "stimulation overload!" I avoided the TV!

To stay mentally active, I reverted to my prior pastime activities. I tried to play cards with Mom and Dad. *New self-discovery* and *variable*—I couldn't follow the sequencing involved! When it was my turn, I had a long delay in processing which card to play. At the end of a hand, adding my cards together was very difficult and tiring. After I had played my "new strenuous mental activity" for ten to twenty minutes, the cognitive fatigue set in. All the new self- and patient-discoveries caused frustration for everyone.

The "why" questions reappeared from the unknown and unseen. Back to . . . Pre-Op Sandra had no difficulty with these tasks. Pre-Op Sandra had stayed up all night to play games and watch television. "What's happening to me?" I would ask. *"Why?"* The unseen answer to the cognitive/mental fatigue finally came to me by way of another analogy.

During my recovery, I personally believe Sally's healing process mimicked that of a marathon runner in training. Therefore, I'm using a marathon runner as the basis for my analogy to help everyone see and understand the cognitive/mental fatigue a TBI survivor might succumb to. It will benefit all involved. The premise of cognitive/mental fatigue is this: *Thinking is your brain running!*

Sally's purpose in training is the same as

that of a physical runner who has experienced a period of immobility. For Sally, her immobility was caused by brain surgery. Now Sally is back in training to successfully run marathons again, to run with the agility and endurance she had before the brain surgery and prior to the years of abusive seizures.

Presurgery and pre-seizures, Sally had been a lifetime marathon runner. "Running" is how I describe the action of mental processing. "Distance" is how I describe the amount/length *of incoming information. So before these events, Sally was running great distances every day. She was always thinking and processing new information.*

Post-surgery, as a runner, Sally had just been through a very traumatic event. She had suffered various dismemberments (resected areas), to say the least. In regard to the cognitive/mental fatigue, Sally is beginning her "post-surgery training." She is in training to "run" (cognitive/mental processing) "marathons" (continuous incoming information) again.

In her training, Sally uses a treadmill to strengthen her endurance. The speed and incline of the treadmill is determined by two factors. First, the amount of information intake *determines the* speed of the treadmill, *and second, the* complexity of information *determines the* incline of the treadmill.

Here are several examples of how this analogy works. Cognitively processing how much two plus two is? The treadmill moves at a walking pace with no incline. Cognitively processing the sum of my eight cards? The treadmill moves at a jogger's pace with a slight incline.

When there is a conversation of any length to cognitively process, the treadmill moves at a runner's pace. The number of people and the depth of information involved determine how steep the incline. To successfully participate in and follow a conversation would be considered, from my personal experience, a workout for an accelerated and healthy runner.

In conclusion regarding this analogy, the survivors' and supporters' "regimen" (mental activity) for the healing brain needs to resemble a physical runner in training after immobility. My regimen, once I solved this riddle, meant that Sally needed to begin slowly. She tired quickly from "exertion." ("Exertion" is how I describe the *function* of cognitive/mental processing.) To accomplish a beneficial exercise regimen, the patients and their supporters *must* be aware of all working factors in just one workout. Let me help you by describing Sally's workout.

> Envision Sally standing on a treadmill. (The treadmill represents the cognitive/mental information itself.) After being immobile for a period of time, Sally is very weak and obese (swollen from surgery).
>
> When Sally is given a piece of information, the treadmill begins to move (incoming information). This forces Sally to move (mental activity). She's trying to move in unison with the treadmill (process the incoming information). If Sally overexerts her abilities (exceeds function) to keep up (processing) with the treadmill (information) and

*doesn't succeed (cognitive disconnect), Sally falls
off the treadmill (overwhelmed) into the abyss of
spiraling emotions.*

Thus, after each workout, Sally is fatigued. She needs to stay idol and rest. Sally, along with all other brains, is only at rest when one sleeps. So after any mental activity, I'd immediately take a nap to allow Sally to rest. When she felt rested, I would wake up. Then Sally would continue with her training. Just like a runner!

Now everyone can see why a patient with TBI will become mentally/cognitively fatigued! Any cognitive processing for a TBI survivor is being active. To the supporters, I beg you to understand the activity and fatigue involved with TBI recovery. Unfortunately, early in my journey, one of the several things I was called was "lazy." Nobody could see my mental activity.

For example, after "working out" for three hours to compose one simple e-mail, Sally needed to rest. After I'd woken up, I was asked, "Hey, lazybones. Are you going to do *anything* today?" *Don't anyone say this to a survivor!* If you have read my analogy, you have no excuse not to understand. Thank you.

To the survivors, I say, "Please don't feel bad or become discouraged from the mental fatigue." It is acceptable to take a rest. You need to. I recall my six-month checkup and telling the neurologist, "I'm tired of being tired!"

His response? "You should be tired. Rest as often as you can."

Good validation. This was one of only a few doctors' orders I haven't defied (yet) during recovery.

In trying to find a positive from resting so often, I noted that I found encouragement when I experienced a conversation lasting a minute longer. Then I could play an extra hand of cards. Therefore, resting more may increase your brain's endurance sooner than if you tried to fight the fatigue. It's all right. You're *not* lazy. Your brain is *healing!*

To help everyone devise their own regimen, I'd like to share something I've implemented in mine. It's the acronym "KISS," standing for "Keep it simple, stupid." When I first heard my supporter, Kim, say it (she uses it in general), I laughed, thinking it was only funny. Then I discovered that saying "KISS" to myself and explaining it to others helped me avoid or overcome the mental running and exertion. This has been very relevant in regard to Sally's training. Perhaps it will be in yours, too. The acronym is not meant to be disrespectful. Find the humor in it.

If you're curious how this acronym can make such an impact in a survivor's recovery, the concept of KISS is simple. As a TBI survivor, don't take on a task that requires more than one or two steps to complete. If you're trying to accomplish something and feel overwhelmed, simplify what you're doing. An example would be making dinner. Instead of cooking a roast in the oven while making several side dishes on the stovetop, put it all in a Crock-Pot. Keep it simple.

For the supporter, don't ask a TBI survivor to do something that takes more than one or two steps. If you see them struggling, help them. Help simplify what they are trying to accomplish. Speaking metaphorically, get the Crock-Pot out of the cabinet for them. Put the contents in together.

During times of frustration, don't be discouraged. Eventually the complexity of tasks will increase. The fatigue will decrease. When the Sallys in recovery are ready, you will feel and see it. Just remember to increase in moderation along the way.

To those who don't know me personally, I might sound hypocritical right now, rambling on about simplicity while I'm writing a book during my recovery. Sure, I've taken on the complex task of processing so much while I'm recovering. Well, I am a complex and stubborn individual. I have never called myself brilliant! I do, however, practice what I recommend to others. I've learned over time how to step back. The only thing I have left to say about this concept is this, "Thanks, Kim! You're so helpful and smart!"

The last discovery in Seattle has remained my own burden . . . *humiliation!* My introduction to humiliation occurred when, after thirty-plus years, I needed my mother's help with dressing, undressing, and getting in and out of the bathtub. Mom also had to wash and dry me because of my physical weakness, imbalance, fatigue, and lack of coordination. I began to feel different about myself. My personal perception started to change when I discovered my inability to handle personal care. Simply put, I felt pathetic, angry, and frustrated.

Even so, I didn't understand what was manifesting these feelings. Was I experiencing humiliation or embarrassment? It took me time to understand that it was humiliation. This is how I decipher the identity of the two. These are my own definitions:

> Embarrassment touches only the surface of your being. It is caused when something affects your outer feelings: sadness, happiness, or shyness. The feeling will dissipate. You're able to forget about it over time.
>
> On most occasions, embarrassment is the result of something accidental. Oops, I didn't mean to say or do that. I or you should have knocked first before entering the bathroom. The encounter with embarrassment is instantaneous. It happens, it's done, and it's later forgotten. Nothing has changed. You personally have not changed.
>
> Humiliation, on the other hand, affects your inner being, who and what you are. It doesn't let go over time. It lingers in your heart and soul, stealing your pride, dignity, and self-worth, making you feel inadequate, the way you do when needing help with personal care. Unlike embarrassment, humiliation occurs because things have changed. You have changed.

I don't wish humiliation on anyone, but unfortunately, it will happen. I've concluded from personal experience and from listening to other TBI survivors that humiliation is a staple in TBI recovery. What I do wish for everyone is that you have someone like my mom to help you through it. Especially in the beginning.

When I began experiencing this new discovery, Mom was great at trying to ease my humiliation and discomfort. She gave no extra attention to the tasks that had me feeling humiliated. She just went with it, using her motherly instincts, thus making me feel less childlike and less of a burden. You were the best nurse, Mom!

Thank you so much! You are the best mom, too!

I encourage other supporters to do the same. Stay relaxed. Do whatever you need to help. Carry it out in a matter-of-fact way. It is what it is.

I previously detested that saying! Whenever I heard it, I always thought it was used as a cop-out. "If you don't like something, then change it!" was my mentality. "Don't settle or surrender to a challenge." Personally, I had to lose some of my brain to understand that "It is what it is" wasn't so bad after all. It's about acceptance, not about weakness or lack of courage. Using my own words, I'd say, "Stress is heavy. Acceptance is uplifting." Now I follow the saying "It is what it is" with "Let's move on."

After several days in the hotel suite, I felt desperate to return home. I needed familiar surroundings, the security of my physical constant. My intention was to leave all the challenges and self-discoveries in Seattle. What I didn't know was that, when leaving the hotel suite, everything I intended to leave behind came with me. I carried my relentless extra baggage on the voyage home.

Chapter 10

Voyage Home

*M*y voyage home began when leaving for the airport, and it didn't begin well. Each acquired challenge continued as I stumbled out of the hotel door and into the taxi. To set the scene, our taxi was over-scented and driven by a very bad driver. The odor was so intense! *Am I experiencing a previous precursor to having a seizure?* I wondered. Fortunately, I was not.

Before getting in, Dad suggested I sit in the front, which would make it easier for me to maneuver in and out. Dad was right about it being easier for me physically. Yes, Dad, I admit you were correct, and it's in writing! Even so, in addition to the horrible nauseating smell, sitting in the front imposed other challenges during the ride to the airport.

The following is something for everyone to keep in mind when traveling after a TBI.

For one, I had an unobstructed view of the surroundings quickly passing by. The VO was horrible. Closing my eyes would have been a logical solution, but I could not. My nausea was worsening from the swaying of the taxi weaving through traffic. When the driver would slow and accelerate rapidly, the pain and pressure inside my skull was fierce! All I could do was wish to arrive at the airport to go home. Like my mom sometimes says, "Be careful what you wish for." Mom, you were right, too!

After our safe arrival at the airport, I had wheelchair assistance. As I was being wheeled inside the terminal, the challenges and variables made sure I didn't forget my extra baggage. I had it all. The vultures were circling above, planning for their next moment of attack. My humiliation was sitting comfortably on my lap for everyone to see! Once inside, my mental reaction to the environment was, *All right, challenges, let the war commence.* It did.

Immediately I was under siege from the overwhelming chaos. People were scattered everywhere. Everyone was moving rapidly in different directions. I felt like a little fish in the open sea. I became a subject in unknown danger. My anxiety, fear, and panic increased.

During my writing, this experience has given me a flashback. It resembles my first scuba dive in the open water. There were a couple of us divers sitting in the rocking boat somewhere on the ocean. I was the first to enter the deep open water. I tipped backward off the boat—and landed in the middle of a large school of swimming jellyfish. In fear, I began my descent to escape the danger they presented—I didn't want anyone having to peepee on me. After the descent, I came face-to-face with a barracuda! This was my first documented experience of having a panic attack.

In the airport, I was reliving an identical sense of exposure to danger. Coming from the center of this liability to injury was so much noise! The busy people were talking and yelling, dragging and dropping their luggage. My auditory and visual overstimulation rapidly increased. To complete the immediate challenges in the airport, the structural layout of this particular one had been confusing before my brain surgery.

Even though I had humiliating wheelchair assistance to help me, I was totally discombobulated on the inside. Sally was bombarded with incoming stimuli. She was trying to process as much of my surroundings as possible. Sally was running as fast as she could. The treadmill was moving at a runner's pace with a very steep incline. Bob was not helpful. He was unable to confirm any of Sally's sparse recalls. From the effects of Bob making the environment ambiguous, Sally's agility and balance was weakening. He was tormenting me as well.

Bob transported me back into my spatial oblivion with "I'm not sure about this place. Maybe it's familiar? Maybe it's not. Are you sure?" Hmm. I just realized something. Did I subconsciously give my nemesis a male name?

Externally, nobody could see what I was going through, either emotionally or mentally. They could only see that I looked empty or "odd." This is how my supporters have described the visual. I had no facial or emotional expressions. Looking in the mirror, I could see that my eyes resembled opaque glass, with my face being unyielding stone. My void stare didn't help in my first public journey. It played into the hands of my challenges and humiliation. They had me fighting on defense.

Going through security, I was asked "the" questions. That introduced me to a new self-discovery. I had a longer processing delay with understanding and answering questions in a public setting. My new discovery of being in public intensified my confusion, anxiety, and panic. For others, my delay caused confusion with skepticism. "She's in a wheelchair, but she looks fine physically. What's wrong with her?" I began to sense each stranger was looking at me differently, as if I had a mark on my forehead (more humiliation).

To help the supporters understand the sensation some of us survivors may feel when in public, I ask you to reflect on these questions. Please. Have you ever had someone give you "the look" that made you check to see if you forgot to put your pants on? Or say to you after you spoke, "What turnip truck did you fall off of?" Have you ever experienced somebody doubting and questioning your every action and inaction? Looking at you with disbelief? Whispering to another . . . "Faker!"

I had a mental sense of these questions and scenarios coming from everyone I came in contact with, either up close or in the distance. Thus, I made another new self-discovery: being in public was diminishing my remaining self-esteem and self-confidence after surgery. Hence, I was not only insecure being outside my comfort zone but also insecure within myself and unsure of my abilities.

So how did I try to cope with my feelings? I focused on making it to Denver for our connecting flight. Why? First, it gave me just *one* objective to focus on, aiding Sally to exercise without obstructive hurdles. Second, I believed I'd have a greater chance with familiarity.

In my previous career, I'd worked for a major airline at Denver International Airport. Therefore, my coping strategy became telling myself that being there would place me in familiar surroundings and I would feel more comfortable, at ease, and grounded. Perhaps I could even make it through the layover without having an unpleasant, surreal feeling. Maybe Bob could finally help Sally by recalling and confirming something. I wanted out of my spatial oblivion!

Eventually we boarded the Denver-bound plane in Seattle. I don't recall any in-flight portion of this leg. Sally needed a long rest after her airport workout! We woke up in Denver when taxiing to the gate. I felt happy and eager to deplane. My coping strategy remained centered around familiarity. I wanted to believe Bob could now confirm what I was close to seeing, finally freeing me from my spatial oblivion, ending the ambiguity, the feeling of being lost, and the self-doubt.

As I was wheeled down the jetway, my palms were clammy. I was so focused on the exit that I forgot to breathe. We finally reached the end. So did my optimism. The environment was filled with haze. My sigh of relief after deplaning turned into a sigh of despair.

My coping strategy didn't produce the outcome I'd hoped for. I felt reintegrated into my spatial oblivion. Most of the environment was unfamiliar. The only familiarity came from the "skeptics" looking at me *again!* While I was wheeled through the concourse, Bob couldn't recall details to confirm where I was physically. Same old Bob. I was lost and panicked. Same "getting old" feeling, although now, I had a new emotional challenge: apprehension.

While I sat in the boarding area, apprehension set in. *Will Bob recall anything after this last leg? Will my physical constant still be there? Or will it be overtaken by my spatial oblivion? Should I not board the plane to preserve what Sally knows about home, to not chance having my constant lost in the unawareness?*

I tried calming myself, tried to give myself hope through reason. My neuropsychologist, Dan, calls it self-talk. (I'm just confirming to the readers that I'm not a nut case.) So I'm talking quietly to myself. "Hold it together, Sandra. You're almost home to your physical constant. You've spent more recent time there than here. You should have no more challenges with familiarity after we leave." With those words, I was wheeled out to our final flight, my extra baggage in tow.

The plane was a small commuter with a turboprop engine. When we reached the stairs, I had to gate-check my walker, which was a gift from the hospital. Unfortunately, I had to be wheeled around all day, so Mom and Dad had been carrying it. Standing up to attempt the stairs was difficult. Even though I'd been sitting all day, I was still physically weak and shaky. It also did not help that my humiliation was still perched on my lap. It didn't want to move. The humiliation wanted to remain with me so that everyone could see it! In addition to the humiliation, as I attempted the stairs, the vultures were circling arrogantly above, unafraid of the propellers and me. I made it safely on board.

The commuter flight to Cody was a whole other challenge! Yep, I was definitely awake during this leg of the voyage. I tried desperately to adapt to the darker, colder, and smaller cabin. The most subtle movements of the aircraft were noticeable, along with the continued humming and vibration of the propellers. This caused intense pressure in my head and more nausea. I did have an unexpected distraction, though.

It was my first experience outside the hospital with seeing and being near individuals in a small, enclosed environment. Inside the plane, there was a man sitting catty-corner from me who looked very familiar. I spent the duration of the flight thinking, Who are you? The answer never came to me. You might wonder why I didn't just ask the man who he was. Simply put, it never occurred to me, but if it had occurred to me, my diminishing self-esteem wouldn't have allowed me to ask.

As the loud, vibrating plane landed, I thought, *I'm only a couple of minutes away from reuniting with my physical constant. Will I be able to sigh with relief this time after deplaning? Will this moment be as I anticipated and hoped? Will I be able to finally ditch the wheelchair and just grab my walker (less humiliation) and go home?*

No . . . no . . . definite no.

My homecoming was delayed. I was asked to wait on board while the other passengers deplaned. As everyone else deplaned, each one had to look at me in passing, and I thought they looked at me with skepticism. Not only was confusion taking place inside my head, there was confusion taking place outside the aircraft and airport doorway. *Oh, great!* My walker had been left on the ramp in Denver. I think the vultures took it!

The apologetic agent brought a wheelchair for me to use (humiliation and frustration). Once inside the airport, my anxiety, panic, and apprehension returned. My spatial oblivion remained. Bob was causing ambiguity.

Everything was either unclear through my eyes or unknown in my spatial memory. There wasn't anything absolute or definite for me. I *knew* there should have been! I was so scared! My mental challenges and insecurities intensified. During the wait for our luggage, I felt trapped inside a hornet's nest.

Many people were gathered around the tiny baggage area. The simultaneous conversations echoed in my head, but I couldn't decipher anything. It sounded like buzzing noise through my ears, bees flying around inside my skull. It caused throbbing head pressure.

Here's a suggestion to supporters: keep TBI survivors away from crowds.

While I was sitting there in my unseen pain, strangers continued to give me "the look" (continued humiliation). My consciousness was screaming, *Is there something to remove this mark on my forehead?* I was successfully containing my emotions—that is, until Dad rightfully asked me a simple question: "Where did you park your car when you flew out?"

Oh my gosh! This simple question triggered an emotional bomb to go off in my head. The internal wall I had spent weeks erecting to contain my emotions began to crumble. I guess after having a very long, stressful, mentally and physically tiring, humiliating, frustrating, overstimulating, nauseating, head-pounding, challenging, disappointing, and self-discovering day, I emotionally imploded! The thick barrier I had built to protect myself from this outcome was quickly demolished. The weight of the rubble gave me a heavy heart.

The crumbling began when I couldn't recall if I'd written down the location of my car or even where I would have placed it if I had written it down. What I knew and what I learned in this moment intensified my frustration. I knew Pre-Op Sandra would have known and done everything precisely. I'd just learned that Post-Op Sandra had little recollection of *anything!*

I vaguely recall answering Dad that I didn't know and to push the alarm button to find it. I clearly recall Mom's response to mine. "Show respect toward your father!" Our whole exchange took place in the midst of everyone (the ultimate humiliation). I truly feel terrible if I showed disrespect toward Dad. Sorry, Dad. Looking back, though, I have to say that Sally did an excellent job of problem solving, only a couple of weeks after brain surgery!

This rationale is not an excuse for acting poorly, if I did. What it is, though, is another example showing that supporters need to keep an open mind. Please remember what the survivor has recently gone through. Try to put yourself and your questions into perspective before asking and reacting. I cannot stress enough that this is not an excuse for my behavior. From a TBI survivor's perspective, it's learning from hindsight about reality. The simplest questions asked by a supporter may not be so simple for a TBI survivor to answer.

My awesome dad was able to find my car. He pulled up to the waiting area where Mom and I were sitting inside. (I was still in a dang wheelchair!) The three of us were eager to end the day's voyage at my house. That was true, until I saw . . . *my* car?

When Dad pulled up, seeing "my car" elicited apprehension. I felt the need to wait a few minutes before getting in. It was unpleasantly cold and windy, but I had to take time to *mentally process* what I was looking at. I could recall the color of my car. I could even recall the name of the make and model. Basically, I could recall what was written on my insurance card. What I was unable to recall, no thanks to Bob, was what my car actually *looked like.*

Mom and Dad were great about giving me a moment. They waited patiently for me to get my bearings. Even though I was physically and mentally tired, I was not going to surrender to my challenges, especially with being so near to the end of my voyage home. Surrendering now would be injustice after fighting the long day's battle. My immediate focus became to "conquer" Bob. I had to confirm that this was my car!

As Mom and Dad were experiencing the Wyoming wind and cold, this is what I was experiencing in trying to defeat Bob's ambiguity.

"Bob, my car is red."

Your last car was red, too!

"Well, my current *car is a four-door hatchback."*

So was your last car!

"My car has the AWD emblem."

So did your last car!

"Bob! My last car was old! *My current one is* new!"

Silence . . . Hah! *I was ready to get in.*

Thankfully, after that exchange, it was too dark to see the interior. I sat in the back this time. I wanted a peaceful ride home. Dad didn't need directions from me, so I closed my eyes for the short ride. My mind was still processing the car experience. Before we were out of the airport parking lot, I became comfortably drawn into talking to my spiritual constant.

Dear Lord, the experience I just went through with seeing my car transformed my eagerness to return to my physical constant into fear. Is what just happened an omen? As to what is waiting for me at home, I'm not sure if I even want to go home or if I'm ready to go home. Please help me, Lord. I do surrender to you . . . to you only!

The next thing I remember is stepping awkwardly into the house through the back door. My home was in complete darkness. The night sky was overcast, so I couldn't see anything inside. This *was* a blessing. From the darkness I received comfort. There was no spatial conflict. My other senses brought familiarity and calmness.

I could smell my home's identity. I could hear the familiarity of the lilac bushes lightly brushing against the windows from outside. Keeping the house dim for me, Mom guided me to the bathroom. While brushing my teeth, I could taste the familiar difference in my tap water. When I was done, she guided me into my bedroom and helped me into bed, my bed! Mom made sure the baby monitor on my nightstand worked. This was in case I needed them during the night. Next, she lovingly tucked me in. Dad came in before she left. We all said our good-nights and our thanks. Our last moments together, on this day, ended with Mom and Dad giving me a gentle, loving kiss on my aching forehead. Thank you, Mom and Dad.

After they left the room, I curled up in a ball with my rosary in hand. I placed it next to my heart. As I lay there in *my* bed, I could feel the familiar touch of my favorite sheets and blanket. Unlike earlier in the day, I now felt placed in a secure cocoon of serenity and familiarity. I began to feel the weight on my heart dissipate.

These were my concluding thoughts to end my voyage home: I thanked my Lord for Mom and Dad, Sonia, the doctors and nurses, and for everyone who had helped me make it home safely. Most importantly, I thanked him for listening to me in the car, along with answering me by having the night sky dark to dim the house upon walking in, thus making the reunion with my physical constant familiar and comforting. The experience was rewarding after the long days of post-op and this challenge-filled day.

As my eyelids grew heavy and my breaths became lighter, I had my last self-discovery before drifting off. It was a conscious revelation that ended a chapter—not solely a chapter in this book, but a chapter in my *life*. For the first time in several years, I was *not afraid to fall asleep!*

Sweet dreams, and may God bless all TBI survivors, their families, and supporters. I feel *very* blessed to have the people I do in my life. I wish the same for you. Amen.